PERFECT HEALTH

THE COMPLETE GUIDE FOR BODY & MIND

FITNESS & SLIMMING

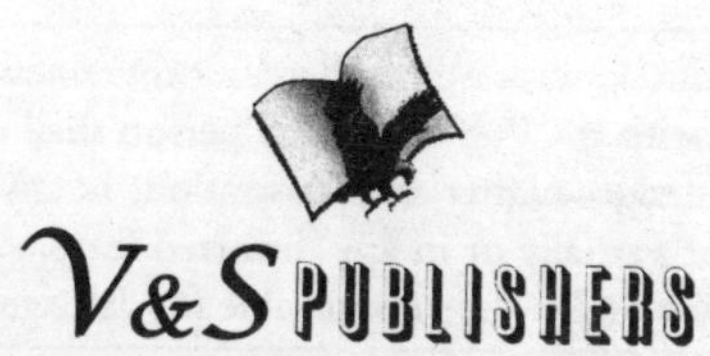

Published by:

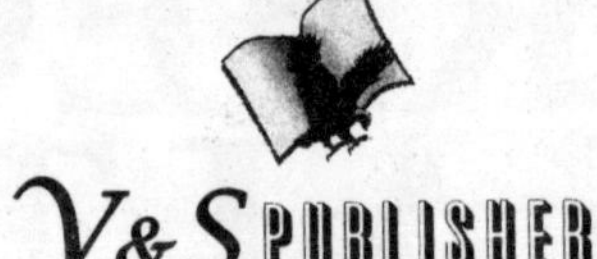

F-2/16, Ansari Road, Daryaganj, New Delhi-110002
011-23240026, 011-23240027 • *Fax:* 011-23240028
Email: info@vspublishers.com • *Website:* www.vspublishers.com

Branch : Hyderabad
5-1-707/1, Brij Bhawan (Beside Central Bank of India Lane)
Bank Street, Koti, Hyderabad - 500 095.
040-24737290.
E-mail: vspublishershyd@gmail.com

ISBN 978-93-815883-7-6

Edition 2014

Printed at : Param Offseters, Okhla, New Delhi-110020

PUBLISHER'S NOTE

According to Francis Bacon, "A healthy body is the greatest chamber of soul; a sick one, its prison." But to maintain a healthy body one must not only follow the rules of moderate health living coupled with a state of moral relaxation exercising one's judgment in meeting the strains and stresses in life but must also understand the disease process, since a proper understanding of not only the health but also of the sickness is essential in maintaining a healthy being.

The present day stress of life produces harmful effects not only on different organs of the body but also on the psyche. There is no denying the fact that both the mind and body are so interlinked that their mutual interaction constitutes equal share in the maintenance of the normal human cycle.

To live a normal healthy life one has to live life and enjoy it. Life can't be a mathematical equation of do's and don't but, put in a judicious manner; the various intricacies of a healthy and diseased body must be well appreciated. If one can understand that the road to healthy living through a life of moderation in one's habit and attitudes towards life, the task becomes much easier.

To make the task easier we present to you *Perfect Health,* a set of four books.

Book I: Perfect Health: Body, Diet & Nutrition
Book II: Perfect Health: Fitness & Slimming
Book III: Perfect Health: Health Hazards & Cure
Book IV: Perfect Health: Stress & Alternative Therapies

This set of four books is not meant to create awareness about the physical well-being alone. There are many books doing that, already. Instead, all the four books are all about creating awareness that fitness of the mind and emotions is as important as the fitness of body. And unless one works at being fit in every way, one is not likely to find true health.

To many, this would seem an unattainable goal but it is not so. The effort required to work towards an integrated health and fitness regime is hardly any more difficult than trying to balance your social and spiritual life. Where there is a will, there is a way. And so with fitness.

Perfect Health provides a complete step-by-step program of mind body medicine tailored to individual needs. The result is a total plan, tailor-made for each individual, to reestablish the body's essential balance with nature; to strengthen the mind-body connection; and to use the power of quantum healing to transcend the ordinary limitations of disease and aging – in short, for achieving perfect health.

CONTENTS

SECTION 1

EXERCISE

Chapter 1

FITNESS

Feeling "fit and fine" is all about fitness. Feeling "fit" pertains to health, and "fine" is about the mental state. Fitness has assumed great significance in the present time because the daily routine of most people is devoid of regular and effective exercise. Our forefathers did not need any gyms or health clubs because their lifestyle involved a lot of physical activity. Walking long distances was a matter of routine; many people used bicycles, which gave them enough exercise. Since there were no televisions, playing outdoor games were their idea of recreation. Women laboured through the day on activities like cleaning, grinding, cooking et al, since there were no fancy gadgets. Unpolluted air, open spaces, unadulterated and fresh food added to their fitness and good health. On the contrary, the present generation has to make an extra effort to get the required physical exercise, the lifestyle has necessitated it.

The very appearance of a person displays his fitness. A fit person has a glow on the face and a good posture. Fitness of the body can be of two kinds - "Organic fitness", generally pertains to a body free of disease and infirmity; in basic terms it means healthy; while "Dynamic fitness" means endurance, flexibility, and strength of the body.

Fitness has an added advantage because the very approach to life changes, resulting in quality life. It brings with it, an optimistic outlook, energetic view and effervescent mind. A fit person can be spotted from a distance because he stands out in a crowd. Need we say more? The advantages of fitness are not unknown and every human being wants to be fit. But most people are on the lookout for easy way out. No wonder most books, newspapers and magazines carry articles on health related issues. The truth is that there are no short cuts to fitness. It is a slow and arduous climb, especially if one is obese and unhealthy.

Fitness Advice

One major factor, which you know, is your diet. Cutting out the sugar is a good idea, although don't think you need to cut it out completely. One must have a lot of fruits and vegetables. A well-rounded diet, with fruits, vegetables, pastas and protein, must be combined with your exercise program to shed those extra pounds. When you travel, when you arrive in a new place try to find restaurants that offer some low-fat meals. Go for a baked potato instead of a burger; even fast-food restaurants are offering salads these days, but leave off the thick dressing.

For meals at home, simple and nutritious food is best. Indulgence once in a while is acceptable provided you don't cheat on your regular meal calories.

As for your exercise programme here are a few things to consider. One, there's no such thing as spot reducing. You can firm up muscles in your stomach, but you'll still need to eliminate more fat from your diet and burn more calories overall to lose weight.

Diet + Exercise = The ideal combination.

The combination of regular exercise and diet offer far more flexibility in achieving negative calorie balance and accompanying fat loss than either exercise or diet alone can. In fact, the addition of exercise to a program of weight control may facilitate a more permanent fat loss so it is wiser not to place total reliance on caloric restriction. Dietary reductions and increase in activity should not be made all at once. Make changes gradually and keep your sights on your goal - a trimmer and healthier you.

Benefits of Regular Exercise

Exercises help to work out the muscles, joints, cardiovascular system, etc, so that when the time comes, normal work can be done without much strain, even in old age. A fit old man can run faster and catch a bus than a younger person when the time comes. No wonder many commercials have this theme to promote their health products. Physical exercises help in increasing blood circulation, provide the muscles with oxygen through the blood streams. All this contributes to greater physical endurance and helps to accomplish daily tasks without much fatigue.

Exercises are the main means of burning calories thereby keeping obesity in check and create a pleasant feeling of fitness. Even if you may not become conscious of it immediately, exercise brings with it an improvement of posture, appearance and self-image. Exercises help to keep the internal organs toned up and perform to their optimum; this in turn helps keep illness away.

Regular and adequate exercise does not guarantee good health and long life, but they certainly help in both. Most people in western countries and now in India die of heart problems, it accounts for almost 65 percent of deaths over the age of 70, and 40 percent deaths over 60 years of age. Exercises help keep the heart if a fit state and people who exercise regularly are less prone to heart ailments in old age.

The Long-term benefit of exercise is that the body is not allowed to gain weight and movement is relatively easier compared to an obese person, and the muscles retain the ability to flex more thereby providing more vigour to the body. This, by itself, is enough to generate the feel good factor.

The hidden benefits of exercising are many, but the main benefit seems to be the ability of the mind to cope up with stress. A fit person laughs more easily and enjoys the very business of living. It is a natural outcome of being fit because it you exercise well, you sleep well, and if you sleep well you remain devoid of stress and fatigue.

Exercise strengthens your heart and trains it to use oxygen more efficiently. As your heart grows stronger, it can pump more blood through your body, which helps your body function. Regular exercise can help keep your arteries more elastic, and build up muscles and bones at the same time. It also keeps you flexible so you can do all the activities you like. Because your muscles need energy to function while exercising, you'll burn calories, which helps you lose weight, lose body fat and gain lean muscles. Exercise can also help speed up you metabolism.

Regular exercise has been shown to decrease the risk of heart disease. It is also known to prevent cancer, obesity, increase flexibility and range of motion, improve mood and stamina, and give an injection of overall energy. In fact, aerobic exercise can also improve your mental health and ability to think, as well as perform and be creative. And if you exercise regularly, it serves as a good model for children: They are more likely to make exercise a habit it they see you doing it. Experts report that by increasing your fitness level even by minimal amounts, you are actually adding years to your life-no matter when you start or what you look like.

Physical activity builds healthy bones, muscles and joints, and reduces the risk of colon cancer. Physical activity also brings psychological benefits. For example, it reduces feelings of depression and anxiety, improves mood and promotes a sense of well-being

Exercise is not just for Olympic hopefuls or supermodels. In fact, you're never too unfit, too young or too old to get started. Regardless of your age, gender or role in life, you can benefit from regular physical activity. If you're committed, exercise in combination with a sensible diet can help provide an overall sense of well-being and can even help prevent chronic illness, disability and premature death.

Benefits of Increased Activity Are:

Improved health

- ❑ Increased efficiency of heart and lungs
- ❑ Reduced cholesterol level
- ❑ Increased muscle strength
- ❑ Reduced blood pressure
- ❑ Reduced risk of major illnesses such as diabetes and heart disease
- ❑ Weight loss

Improved sense of well-being

- ❑ More energy
- ❑ Less stress
- ❑ Improved quality of sleep
- ❑ Improved ability to cope with stress
- ❑ Increased mental acuity

Improved appearance

- ❑ Weight loss
- ❑ Toned muscles
- ❑ Improved posture

Enhanced social life

- ❑ Improved self-image
- ❑ Increased opportunities to make new friends
- ❑ Increased opportunities to share an activity with friends or family members

Increased stamina

- ❑ Increased productivity
- ❑ Increased physical capabilities
- ❑ Less frequent injuries
- ❑ Improved immunity to minor illnesses

Types of Exercises

Exercises can broadly be classified into two main categories, i.e., isometric and dynamic. Isometric exercises are those, when there is muscle activity without much body movement. Examples of these are weight lifting, rowing, etc. Dynamic exercises are those in which muscle movement is achieved through body movement. Playing a game of hockey, football and running are examples of dynamic exercises. Dynamic exercises improve general physical fitness and these are the exercises to be resorted to. The most common types of dynamic exercises are aerobics, running, sports and a variety of indoor exercises.

Who can Exercise?

Anyone can get fitter or a fit person can continue to remain fit. Neither a late start nor a low starting point will completely

deny the benefits of physical fitness. Indeed, a low base offers most individuals a greater potential for improvement. You may never run four-or-five-minute a mile, but what matters is coming close to your own body's potential. The long-term health hazards of not exercising exceed the short-term risks associated with a planned fitness program. But before starting a fitness program, you should be sensible and satisfy yourself that although out of condition and unfit, the exercise will not cause you undue distress.

Time to Exercise

There is no set time that has been or can be laid out for exercises. The time is one that is convenient to the person himself. The only restriction is that one should not exercise when ill or till an hour after meal. Early morning is considered best as this is the time when the air is fresh, the dust levels are low and if you are in a city, the sound levels are also low.

Studies have suggested the body functions more efficiently at different times of the day. Some reports, for instance, have shown that the body's processes are slowest in the morning. Others have found that in the afternoon, strength and aerobic capacity are greatest, suggesting that it might be best to exercise at this time. However, there are two basic principles to exercise that are even more important: If you're both consistent and patient with your training, you'll reap the benefits.

Pollution is heavier in the afternoon, which may affect your breathing. So running, cycling and other outdoor activities done in the early morning or after the evening rush hour may be better. The hot afternoon sun may also be a factor that makes early morning or evening exercise a better choice. So if exercising at night works best because you work full-time, it would be just right for you.

Clothing during Exercise

All exercise clothing should be loose-fitting to permit freedom of movement, and should make the wearer feel comfortable and self-assured. As a general rule, you should wear light clothes than temperatures might indicate. Exercise generates body heat. Light-colour clothing that reflects the sun's rays is cooler in the summer, and dark clothes are warmer in winter. When the weather is very cold, it's better to wear several layers of light clothing than one or two heavy layers. The extra layers help trap heat, and it's easy to shed one of them if you become too warm.

In cold weather, and in hot, sunny weather, it's a good idea to wear something on your head. Wool caps are recommended for winter wears, and some form of tennis or sailor's hat that provides shade and can be soaked in water is good for summer. Never wear rubberised or plastic clothing. Such garments interfere with the evaporation of perspiration and can cause body temperature to rise to dangerous levels.

Set Goals

There are a couple of things you should consider as you embark upon your fitness journey: what are you goals, what are your likes, and how can you best equip yourself to meet your goals?

People exercise for many reasons: to lose weight, to tone their bodies, for their overall health and prevention of serious diseases, for the social aspect of interacting with others or to get out and explore the world. Fitness raises self-esteem and pride in oneself, so a lot of people strive for fitness to achieve these targets. And to meet those goals, you should be able to say what you're hoping to get out of exercise; that way, you'll be more likely to stick to your plan.

Establish Preferences

The best part about exercise is that you can get it in so many ways. Just think about the activities you enjoy, and figure out how you can incorporate them into a workout routine. If you're unfamiliar with the variety of activities you can do, ask the trainers at your gym or friends who have been active longer than you have, for some ideas. One thing to keep in mind: just because your friend likes an activity doesn't mean it is for you. So, take your time to see what's out there and what you'd like to try. You have so many options; why not try them all until you find the exercise plan that suits you best.

Know the Basics

Physical fitness is most easily understood by examining its various components, or "parts." There are basically the following components:

- **Cardio respiratory endurance** – It is the ability to deliver oxygen and nutrients to tissues, and to remove wastes, over sustained periods of time. Long runs and swims are among the methods employed in measuring this component.
- **Muscular strength** – The ability of a muscle to exert force for a brief period of time. Upper-body strength, for example, can be measured by various weight-lifting exercises.
- **Muscular endurance** – It is the ability of a muscle, or a group of muscles, to sustain repeated contractions or to continue applying force against a fixed object. Push-ups are often used to test endurance of arm and shoulder muscles.
- **Flexibility** – It is the ability to move joints and use muscles through their full range of motion. The sit-and-reach test is a good measure of flexibility of the lower back and backs of the upper legs.
- **Body composition** – It is often considered a component of fitness. It refers to the makeup of the body in terms of lean mass (muscle, bone, vital tissue and organs) and fat mass. An optimal ratio of fat to lean mass is an indication of fitness, and the right types of exercise will help you decrease body fat and increase or maintain muscle mass.

What is Cardio?

The term cardiovascular system refers to your heart and blood vessels, which carry oxygen and other nutrients throughout your body. The heart is actually a muscle, and like any other muscle, you can strengthen it with exercise.

If you're breathing hard and can feel your heart beating (and you don't stop), you're doing cardio. Walking, hiking, running, jogging and cycling are some popular examples. Variety is the spice of life. It's easy to tire of the same workout week after week, so it is a good idea to vary it. Besides, varying your workout helps develop and strengthen different muscles and keeps you motivated.

Technically, cardiovascular exercise is any activity that:

- Uses large muscle groups (such as your legs).
- Is rhythmic (you repeat the same basic movements).
- Is aerobic (you take in and use more oxygen than usual).
- Is sustained (you do it for several minutes at a time).

Benefits

Exercise can help to reduce or eliminate some of these risk factors:

- **High blood pressure** - Regular exercise is associated with lower blood pressure.
- **Cigarette smoking** - Smokers who exercise vigorously and regularly are more likely to cut down or stop smoking.
- **Diabetes** - People at their ideal weight are much less likely to develop diabetes. Exercise may also decrease a diabetic's insulin requirements. Exercise can help people lose excess fat or stay at a reasonable weight.
- **Low levels of HDL** - Low levels of HDL (one of the cholesterol-carrying proteins in the blood) have been linked to an increased risk of coronary artery disease. Recent studies have shown that regular physical activity significantly increases HDL levels, and thus reduces your risk.

When not to Exercise?

- Moderate to severe coronary heart disease that causes chest pain from inimical activity.
- A recent heart attack. A three-month waiting period is considered standard before moderate; medically supervised exercise programme can begin.
- Severe heart valve defects and heart beat irregularities.

- A greatly enlarged heart and certain type of congenital heart disease.
- Uncontrolled diabetes where you blood sugar levels fluctuate constantly.
- High blood pressure not controlled by medication.
- Any infectious disease during its acute stage.

When to Consult a Doctor?

- If you have a heart condition or you've had a stroke, and the doctor recommended only medically supervised physical activity.
- During or right after you exercise, if you often have pains or pressure in the left or mid-chest area, left neck, shoulder or arm.
- You've developed chest pain within the last month.
- If you tend to lose consciousness or fall over due to dizziness, or you feel extremely breathless after mild exertion.
- If your doctor has recommended that you take medicine for your blood pressure, heart condition or for stroke.
- If your doctor says you have bone, joint or muscle problems that could be made worse by the proposed physical activity.
- If your medical condition or other physical reason not mentioned here that might need special attention in an exercise program, i.e. insulin-dependent diabetes.
- If you are middle-aged or older, haven't been physically active, and plan a relatively vigorous exercise programme.

If none of these is true for you, you can start on a gradual, sensible programme of increased activity tailored to your needs. If you feel any of the physical symptoms listed above when you start your exercise programme, contact your doctor right away. If one or more of the above affect you, an exercise-stress test may be used to help plan an exercise programme.

Exercise and Weight Loss

All agree that physical activity is related to fat loss and sustained weight control. The difference between overweight and normal weight is not solely a product of caloric intake. It is also a result of physical activity levels. Sedentary lifestyle is a prime cause of chronic obesity. Exercise not only control weight, but also regular exercise promotes numerous health benefits and is a significant factor in improving your overall health and fitness levels.

One is the belief that housework or "running around the office" constitutes exercise. People are often fatigued at the end of the day and think that this is evidence of an active life. However, for most people that tired feeling comes from mental not physical exertion. Another myth is the belief that certain exercises can burn fat from specific parts of the body. "Spot reduction" simply cannot take place. Specific, localised exercises are great for improving muscle tone but they do not reduce fat.

Mobilization of fat during selective exercise is not restricted to the underlying fatty tissue of that body part. The fat on top of the muscle belongs to the whole body and fat stores will only be burned if the total energy expenditure is greater than energy input. While all physical activity is beneficial, cardiovascular or aerobic exercise is most effective in promoting weight loss and sustained weight control.

Before Beginning a Regimen

There are some facts that one must know before one begins any kind of exercise regimen. The process of warming up, stretching, loosening of the muscles and finally the cooling down after the exercise is a very important. Failing to observe these rules can actually land you in deep trouble and muscle injury.

Warm-up/Cool Down

Before you begin bicycling, walking or running, whether indoors or outside, do some deep massage to your whole knee area. That means above and below, front and back of the knee. Then some deep massage your lower back and ankle areas. Begin your workout slowly. Use good posture and technique. As your body warms up, let your pace rise with it. When it seems that you are ready to really pick up your pace, stop and do some stretching. Then get back to the pace you had just before you stopped.

Do whatever workout you had planned but before the end gradually, bringing your pace down. When you finish your workout it is the best time for a relaxing set of stretches. Lie down on a padded floor mat and put your legs up against a wall for a few minutes, taking this time to relax and recoup. For weight lifting routines, an aerobic workout such as 15-20 minutes on an exercise bike before lifting. Start slowly and pick-up the pace gradually so that at the end of 20 minutes, you are riding pretty seriously.

Standing out of the seat a few times while pedalling during the ride will help stretch some muscles and get the upper body involved. We guarantee you that you will have your best lifting workouts ever! After lifting, do some gentle stretching on a padded floor mat and if you have the time, a few minutes on a treadmill or exercise bike will help flush the garbage out of your muscles. The basics of warming-up and cooling-down are lifelong rules that will keep you from undue muscle strain. Remember that the heart is a muscle too and that it is protected by this warm-up and cool down rules.

Stretching

Stretching helps lengthen the working areas of the muscle, allowing for greater work capacity. So as long as your flexibility is balanced and you are stretching intelligently, the more flexible you are the better. The same goes with strength. So long as you have developed strength over a long period of time and have strength in all areas of your body, you can't be too strong. Stretching should be a lifelong habit rather than just something you do in conjunction with a workout.

In preparation for most sports, some prefer to get massage their muscles before they begin, then after a bit of their workout, stop to stretch and continue with the activity. Your goal should be to have good flexibility and symmetry top to bottom, and front to back. There are specific stretches for specific activities. Stretching in one muscle has an effect on the muscles around it. So, put some thought into how and why you are stretching. Stretching as it relates to lifestyle will help us retain and increase our range of motion, making us more capable of doing many activities throughout our lives.

Loosening up Exercise

These exercises are very necessary before undertaking up strenuous exercises or sport activity, which demand a lot of stress and endurance for prolonged periods.

- **Head circling** - Stand erect with both feet comfortably apart. Place hands on the hips. Pull down chin and look down, circle or rotate the head in one direction 10 times, and then again 10 times in the opposite direction.
- **Arm circling** - Stand erect with legs comfortably apart and hands on both sides. Raise the hands from the front upwards, and bring them down to the sides again from the rear without bending the elbows. Do this 10 times in one direction and then in the other direction.
- **Trunk twisting** - Stand erect with legs comfortably apart and hands at the side. Turn from the trunk upwards to the left and then to the right without lifting the feet off the ground. Repeat the whole exercise 10 times each side.
- **Knee clasping** - Stand erect with legs comfortably apart and hands to the side. Lift one knee bent to the chest. Clasp the knee with both hands and pull towards the chest with pressure. Repeat this 10 times with each knee.
- **Toe touch** - Stand erect with legs comfortably apart. Bend forward without bending the legs to touch the toes with the fingers, and then return to upright position again. Repeat this ten times.

The kinds of exercises you choose must depend on your physical ability as well as your preferences. The most important rule is to choose activities that you enjoy and that are accessible and feasible for you to do regularly. You also should consider whether you want to make your exercise routine during personal time in which you can be alone with your thoughts or a more social activity. Some people find that exercising with others, provide them with support and encouragement and it can even be fun!

Before you begin an exercise programme, you should have a physical examination. If you are over the age of forty, your doctor will probably want to do a stress electrocardiogram to determine how much activity your heart can handle. If you have not exercised regularly for some time, begin slowly with low-impact exercise and gradually increase your activity. If you experience any adverse side effects, such as dizziness, cramps, or chest pain, stop exercising and consult your physician.

Aerobic and Anaerobic Exercises

There are two types of exercise that perform different functions. Aerobic exercise is sustained activity involving the major muscle groups, such as swimming, running, or brisk walking. The heart and respiratory rate increase, and more oxygen is circulated through the body. This kind of exercise strengthens your cardiovascular system and increases your overall strength and stamina. The goal of aerobic exercise is for your pulse to reach a training rate that is appropriate for your age. You must stay at the rate for twenty minutes, and exercise three times a week, in order to reap the benefits of aerobic exercise.

You've probably heard of "low-impact," or anaerobic, exercise. This means that you are not exercising vigorously or long enough to reach and maintain your training heart rate. It does not mean, however, that low-impact exercise is useless. It improves your muscle strength and flexibility and can still be a good outlet for negative feelings that you might have bottled up.

Three kinds of Anaerobic Exercises:

1. **Isotonics** require that your muscles contract against a resistant object with movement, such as in weight lifting.
2. **Isometrics** requires that your muscles contract against resistance, without movement. Instead of building

muscle mass, as in isotonics, isometric exercises simply increase strength without building bulk.

3. **Calisthenics** are stretching exercises, such as sit-ups, toe-touches, and knee-bends. They help increase flexibility and joint mobility.

Strength training

Strength is fundamental for fitness. Even if you are not going to he an Olympic athlete loss of strength leads to back problems and increased risk of injuries, diminishes co-ordination, reduces endurance and promotes fatigue. Body contours change and you begin to feel old before your time. Muscular strength can be regained at any age.

It is never too late – Once you regain strength, it can be sustained with far less effort you took to acquire it. You cannot increase the number of muscle fibres as these are fixed at birth but you can increase their activation levels and muscle bulk.

What is Aerobics?

"Aerobic" means exercising with oxygen. It comprises all activities that cause the heart and lungs to process oxygen at a steady rate over a sustained period of time. It involves exercising large muscle groups for a continuous period and is the most effective way of increasing calorie loss. Oxygen consumption is directly related to the amount of energy being expended, hence the more aerobic the activity, the more calories that will be burned. It is simply exercise that makes the muscles work hard, but not too hard that the heart and lungs cannot keep up with the oxygen demand. For this reason, aerobic exercise must be performed continuously and steadily, allowing for an increased heart rate to be sustained for an extended period.

To reap maximum benefit from aerobic exercise, you have to be working within your training zone, that is, any continuous activity that pushes your heart rate up to between 60% and 90% of the maximum rate for your age.

Aerobic exercise need not be hard and tough exercise; in fact it is not advisable to push yourself too hard, although you do need to make some physical effort to derive any benefit. Aim to build up the level of activity gradually. Once you start to become aerobically fit, you will find your exercise sessions less tiring and your normal day far less exhausting in general. You should aim for between 20 and 60 minutes on three to five days of the week for optimum fitness. This should be done at between 60% and 90% of your normal maximum heart rate.

There are three main criteria that must be fulfilled for aerobic exercise to be complete.

1. The exercises must involve large muscle groups of the body, i.e. the legs in continuous rhythmic motion.
2. The exercises must be continuous for a minimum of twenty to thirty minutes at least thrice a week.
3. It must be vigorous and strenuous for the whole body.

Types of Aerobic Exercises

There are two types of aerobic exercises, low-impact and high-impact aerobic exercises. Both involve similar kinds of exercises, but high-impact aerobics classes provide better cardiovascular exercise. A workout of 30 and 50 minutes designed to work on various parts of the body is the most beneficial type of calorie burner.

What does Typical Aerobics Include?

Jogging/running on the sport, jumping up and down, upper body work using dumbbells and bars, waist twists, lower body work, including squatting, leg and calf raises, star jumps, lunges, kicks, sit ups and bottom crunches.

The aim is to keep on the move for most of the time. Music is an integral part of any aerobics session; it helps to motivate, keep up or vary the pace and makes the workout more lively and enjoyable. You can, of course, play your own choice of music with a rhythm to match, at home.

Rope jumping or skipping is one of the best aerobic exercises. It is a very vigorous form of exercise, which raises heart beat rate, builds strength, improves balance and co-ordination, and increases endurance. The clothes should be loose and comfortable, the floor should not be hard and the area should be well ventilated, preferable an open area if possible. " Skipping produces the greatest fitness in the least possible time". 10 minutes of skipping is equal to 30 minutes on the road.

Aerobic dancing works out more strenuous than most exercises. When it is performed to the beat of music, it becomes enjoyable, more enjoyable if done in a group. Becoming a member of a group or a club can be a good motivator. Classrooms, open areas, locker rooms and such areas encourage interaction with like-minded people with similar goals and can act as a very good motivator. Organised forums have many other facilities to monitor progress, such as counsellors, who recommend the type of exercise, diet and other related issues.

An aerobic exercise is necessary for utilising fat for energy and improving overall fitness levels. It is also essential for improving cardiovascular and respiratory efficiency i.e. the functioning of the heart and lungs. The type of aerobic activity you choose should be based upon your personal preferences and your physical limitations. You could also try mixing it up and select two to three different forms of aerobic exercises.

S.No	Sport	Endurance	Strength	Mobility
1.	Badminton	Good	Good	Good
2.	Basket Ball	Excellent	Good	Good
3.	Boxing	Excellent	Excellent	Normal
4.	Climbing Stairs	Good	Good	Excellent
5.	Cricket	Normal	Normal	Good
6.	Speed Cycling	Excellent	Good	Normal
7.	Dancing	Good	Normal	Normal
8.	Driving	Normal	Normal	Normal

S.No	Sport	Endurance	Strength	Mobility
9.	Football	Good	Good	Good
10.	Golf	Normal	Normal	Good
11.	Gymnastics	Normal	Good	Good
12.	Hockey	Good	Good	Good
13.	Karate	Normal	Good	Good
14.	Running	Excellent	Good	Good
15.	Squash	Good	Good	Excellent
16.	Swimming	Excellent	Excellent	Excellent
17.	Tennis	Good	Good	Good
18.	Volleyball	Normal	Normal	Good
19.	Walking	Good	Normal	Normal
20.	Wrestling	Good	Excellent	Good

Chapter **2**

TARGET HEART RATE

Healthcare professionals recognize the importance of pacing your efforts when you exercise. The goal is not to tire quickly, but still earn the benefit of being physically active. Pacing yourself is especially important if you've been inactive.

What is Heart Rate

Your heart rate is your pulse i.e. the number of times your heart beats in one minute. You can measure your pulse anytime by placing your index and middle fingers on your larynx and sliding them to one side of your neck. Count the number of beats for one minute; that's your pulse.

The important thing to remember about your heart rate is that if you overexert or under-exert yourself, you won't get the best results from you exercise. Regardless of the activity you participate in, if you keep your heart rate between 65 and 80 percent, you're exercising at a good rate. Target heart rates are effective in measuring initial fitness level and monitoring progress after you begin a fitness programme. This approach requires measuring your pulse periodically as you exercise and staying within 50 to 75 percent of your maximum heart rate. This range is called your target heart rate.

Determine Target Heart Rate

Subtract your age in years from 220. This provides the maximum number of heartbeats per minute expected for someone your age. For example, if you were 30 years old, then the target heart rate would be 220 - 30 = 190.

To find the proper exercise intensity zone, multiply the result by the lower and upper limits of your ideal range. If you were after a great cardio workout, you'd multiply your maximum heart rate (our example is 190) by 0.65 to get your lower limit (124). Then you'd multiply your maximum heart rate by 0.80 to calculate the upper limit (152). To monitor your heart rate during your workout, put two fingers on the carotid artery (on either side of your neck), count the beats during a six-second period and add a zero to the count to get your heart rate per minute. It should fall within your lower and upper limits (124 and 152).

Age	Target HR 50-75 %	Zone Average Maximum Heart Rate 100 %
20 years	100-150 beats per minute	200
25 years	98-146 beats per minute	195
30 years	95-142 beats per minute	190
35 years	93-138 beats per minute	185
40 years	90-135 beats per minute	180
45 years	88-131 beats per minute	175
50 years	85-127 beats per minute	170
55 years	83-123 beats per minute	165
60 years	80-120 beats per minute	160
65 years	78-116 beats per minute	155
70 years	75-113 beats per minute	150

Your maximum heart rate is about 220 minus your age. The figures above are averages and should be used as general guidelines.

Alternative to Target Heart Rate

Some people can't measure their pulse or don't want to take their pulse when exercising. If this is true for you, an option is to use a "conversational pace" to monitor your efforts if you're doing moderate activities like walking. If you can talk and walk at the same time, you aren't working too hard. If you can sing and maintain your level of effort, you're probably not working hard enough. If you get out of breath quickly, you're probably working too hard, especially if you have to stop and catch your breath.

When to use the Target Heart Rate

If you want to participate in more vigorous activities like brisk walking and jogging, where the "conversational pace" approach may not work, then try using the target heart rate. It works for many people, and it's a good way for healthcare professionals to monitor your progress.

How do Heart Rate Monitors Help

Whether you are just starting a biking programme or are a seasoned veteran, a heart rate monitor can be the perfect complement to your biking or fitness programme. A heart rate monitor, like a speedometer, tells you how hard your heart is working (in beats per minute) during indoor or outdoor workouts. By working in the target heart rate zone you can make the most of every workout without ever over-doing it.

Heart rate monitors provide improved accuracy for measuring exercise intensity measurable results, to help keep you motivated. An automatic and convenient way to monitor heart rate and track results increases safety because monitors help to avoid over-exertion. Continuous feedback helps you in continuing your workout, in the proper target heart rate zone.

Gradual Stepup

When starting an exercise programme, aim at the lowest part of your target zone (50 percent) during the first few weeks. Gradually build up to the higher part of your target zone (75 percent). After six months or more of regular exercise, you might be able to exercise comfortably up to 85 percent of your maximum heart rate, if you wish - but you don't have to exercise that hard to stay in condition.

How Many Times a Week

Exercise should be done at least five days consecutively, each week. The human body craves consistency and can make adjustments to long-term demands placed upon it. If you exercise three times per week, it will have a conditioning effect on your heart, but the heart is not the only thing that needs to perform efficiently during exercise. The other organs and muscle tissues will respond much differently to five days in a row. For five days in a row, the body continues to receive the message that it needs to perform efficiently in order to keep up. It adjusts to meet the demand and the result is efficient operation of the whole system, all the time, even on the two days you don't exercise.

Five days of regular, vigorous exercise does stimulate efficiency throughout the body. Too much vigorous exercise can cause the body to go into the survival mode and cause damage to the regular efficient system. This is why it is vital that exercise is begun gradually and increased gradually.

How can physical activity or exercise help condition the body?

Some activities improve flexibility, some build muscular strength and some increase endurance. Some forms of continuous activities involve using the large muscles in your arms or legs, called endurance or aerobic exercises. They benefit the heart because they make it work more efficiently during exercise and at rest. Brisk walking, jumping rope, jogging, bicycling, cross-country running and dancing are examples of aerobic exercises that increase endurance.

Improving Physical Fitness

Programs designed to improve physical fitness take into account frequency (how often), intensity (how hard), and time (how long), and provide the best conditioning.

The FIT Formula:

F = frequency (days per week)
I = intensity (how hard, e.g., easy, moderate, vigorous) or percent of heart rate
T = time (amount for each session or day)

Fitness Formula

If you're interested in improving your overall conditioning, health experts recommend that you should get at least 30 minutes of moderately intense physical activity on all or most days of the week. Examples of moderate activity include brisk walking, cycling, swimming or doing home repairs or yard work. If you can't get in 30 minutes all at once, aim for shorter bouts of activity (at least 10 minutes) that add up to half hour per day.

Instead of thinking in terms of a specific exercise programme, work toward permanently changing your lifestyle to incorporate more activity. Remember that muscles used in any activity, any time of day, contribute to fitness.

FIT for Healthy People

For health benefits to the heart, lungs and circulation, perform any vigorous activity for at least 30 -60 minutes, 3 - 4 days each week at 50 - 75 percent of your maximum heart rate. Moderate -intensity physical activities for 30 minutes or longer on most days, provide some benefits. Physical activity need not be strenuous to bring health benefits. What's important is to include activity as part of a regular routine.

Activities that are especially beneficial when performed regularly include brisk walking, hiking, and stair climbing, aerobic exercise, jogging, running, bicycling, rowing, swimming, and such activities such as soccer and basketball that include continuous running.

The training effects of such activities are most apparent when exercise intensities exceed 50 percent of a person's maximum heart rate. Adults who maintain a regular routine of physical activity of longer duration or greater intensity are likely to have greater benefits. However, physical activity should not be overdone. Too much exercise can result in muscle soreness and a higher risk of injury. For people who can't exercise vigorously or who are sedentary, scientific evidence supports the notion that even moderate-intensity activities, when performed daily, can have long-term health benefits. These activities help lower the risk of cardiovascular diseases. Such activities include walking for pleasure, gardening, housework, dancing and prescribed home exercise. They also include recreational activities such as tennis, badminton, soccer, basketball and touch football.

Terms of Fitness

A well-conditioned body has the following attributes:

1. **Cardio-vascular fitness** - That means that your heart is fit.
2. **Cardio-respiratory fitness** - This means that your lungs are in good shape.
3. **Flexibility** - This means that you can move your body in a full range of motion easily like when you were younger.
4. **Endurance** - This means that your muscles can do something over before reaching fatigue. Endurance gets better when cardio-vascular fitness combines with strength.

Opting for the Right Exercise

The keys to selecting the right kinds of exercise for developing and maintaining each of the basic components of fitness are found in these principles:

- **Specificity** - pick the right kind of activities to influence each component. Strength training results in specific strength changes. Also, train for the specific activity you're interested in. For example, optimal swimming performance is best achieved when the muscles involved in swimming are trained for the movements required. It does not necessarily follow that a good runner is a good swimmer.
- **Overload** - work hard enough, at levels that are vigorous and long enough to overload your body above its resting level, to bring about improvement.

- ❑ **Regularity** - you can't hide physical fitness. At least three balanced workouts a week are necessary to maintain a desirable level of fitness.
- ❑ **Progression** - increase the intensity, frequency and/ or duration of activity over periods of time in order to improve.

Some activities can be used to fulfill more than one of your basic exercise requirements. For example, in addition to increasing cardio respiratory endurance, running builds muscular endurance in the legs, and swimming develops the arm, shoulder and chest muscles. If you select the proper activities, it is possible to fit parts of your muscular endurance workout into your cardio respiratory workout and save time.

Chapter **3**

YOGA

Why to do Yoga

There are many options with which you can profitably engage your free time. You want to exercise, why not a gym or a health club? You could build a rock- solid body, trim your buttocks, flatten your tummy and be ready for the beach. Maybe you just want to relax, let go, and unwind. Life has enough stress without committing to something else. You could opt for a movie, go out for a meal, or visit some friends. The beauty of doing yoga is that it combines stress relief along with body fitness.

Yoga is viewed as many things by different people. The average person thinks yoga is just stretching exercises for bad backs, stress and tension. Yoga is much more. The exercises or 'asanas' are many and varied, as are the tasks, which they can accomplish. Some of the exercises help to make the body stronger, more flexible and healthier. Others reduce stress and tension and help you to better cope with the trials of everyday life.

Developing your intuition and clear insight is the purpose of other yoga exercises. The underlying purpose of all of the yoga tools is spiritual evolution, the lifting of our consciousness from a mundane, worldly level to an awareness and sensitivity for all creation. Yoga benefits your whole body. Through a systematic set of stretching and strengthening exercises you can stretch and strengthen all of your major muscles groups and develop muscle tone and flexibility. The strengthening of the muscles around the spine is particularly important for keeping the spine in proper alignment and having a healthy, strong spine.

Yoga exercises improve your cardio-vascular system by a strengthening and stretching of the heart muscles and making the arteries and veins more elastic. This elasticity allows the vascular walls to expand and carry more volume of blood to get to the part of the body where it is needed without having to increase the blood pressure. By bending and twisting the body in a myriad of ways, your internal organs get massaged which increases their circulation bringing with the extra blood supply more oxygen and nutrients and taking away with the venous blood flow more toxins and waste material. Similarly, through the bending, twisting, and stretching, you enhance the function of your lymphatic system.

Some yoga exercises improve your eyes, making the eyes healthier, and even help to tone the muscles behind the eyes, which control the shape of the eyes and affect your vision. Through regular practice of yoga postures, your body will regain some of its youth and vigour, making you feel and look younger. You will have more energy and endurance.

Yogic exercises offer a variety of methods for a variety of needs. If you are interested in the just the physical, the mental, the spiritual or all three, yoga works. Yoga is a very effective way of getting fit and healthy, and remaining so. It has its origin in India. The word Yoga means 'communication'. Yoga is a pragmatic science, which has evolved over the years and deals with physical, moral, mental and spiritual well-being. There are eight limbs of Yoga as given out by Patanjali in about 200 B.C. These are as follows :-

Yama - Moral commandments.
Niyama - Purification through discipline.
Pranayama - Rhythmic control of the breath.
Asanas - Postures, which keep the body healthy and strong.
Pratyahara - Freeing the mind from the senses.
Dharana - Concentration.
Dhyana - Meditation.
Samadhi - A state of super consciousness brought about by deep meditation.

The first two control passion and emotion. Pranayama and Pratyahara are known as the inner quest. The last two allow the yogi to realise his 'self'. The relaxation and physical benefits achieved from practising even just once a week are sufficient a reward for many beginners and quickly become apparent.

Fitness through Yoga

Stress, fatigue, depression, obesity and heart troubles are some of the most common offshoots of modern lifestyles. India had an answer to the disorders riddling both the mind and the body thousands of years ago in the form of Yoga. So, yoga is a sure fire way to maintain a high level of fitness in the modern day.

Benefits of Yoga

- Regular practice of yoga strengthens the muscles. Yoga controls cholesterol level, reduces weight, keeps blood pressure under check and improves the functioning of the heart.
- Exercises like the Surya Namaskar improve the capacity of the lungs and oxygenate the blood.
- Stretching and bending during the asanas helps in removing hypertension and ensure better functioning of the nervous system.
- Yoga reduces the process of cell deterioration and delays the ageing process.

Surya Namaskar

Although yoga is a vast subject which works both for mental and physical fitness, if you are targeting physical fitness and do not have the time for a range of asanas, surya namaskar is the regimen for you.

'Surya Namaskar' or salutations to the Sun God is a series of 12 postures that can be performed as one complete exercise. The 'Surya Namaskar' is one of the most comprehensive and basic yogasanas and can be performed every morning or evening or at any convenient time of the day. The exercises stretch and flex the different parts of the body, remove stress, and improve blood circulation.

The Asanas (Postures):

1. **Namaskarasana:** Stand erect facing the sun, with your palms pressed together against the chest in the namaskar posture. The elbows should be level with the shoulders, and the feet close together. Breathe deeply and relax. This posture is good for the stomach muscles.
2. **Urdhva namaskarasana:** Inhale, and raise your arms high above your head, with palms still together and eyes following the hands. Bend your body backwards slowly. This asana stretches the front of your body, relaxes muscles, and improves circulation.
3. **Uttanasana:** Exhale slowly, bend your body forward, and bring your hands down to the ground in a wide arc. Your head should touch the knees. With practice, you should be able to rest your palms fully on the ground. This asana helps in stretching the back, shoulders and hamstrings.
4. **Ekapaada prasaranaasana:** While inhaling, gradually lower the body, raise the head, and move the right leg far back in a wide arc. At the end, the right foot and knee touch the ground, while the left foot remains between the hands. This movement exercises the chest, lower back and legs.
5. **Dwipaada prasaranaasana:** As you exhale, extend the left foot and place it next to the right foot. Keep your arms and body straight, and your eyes looking ahead. In this position, you are resting on your hands and toes.
6. **Bhujangasana:** While inhaling, slowly lower your hips till they are just above the ground. Bend your head and torso as far back as possible. This posture is very good for the spine.
7. **Ashtaanga namaskarasana:** While exhaling, slowly lower your body until only the feet, knees, hands, chest and forehead touch the ground. Maintain the posture for a few seconds. Exercises the shoulders, back and chest.
8. **Bhujangasana:** This is somewhat similar to the position in step 6. While inhaling, with hands and feet on

the ground, pull your body forward and bend it as far back as you can. Exercises the shoulders, lower back, abdomen and hands.

9. **Adhomukha shvaanasana:** As you exhale, curve your body away from the ground. Keep your arms straight, shoulders back, raise your back and hips, and bend your head towards your chest. Exercises the neck, back, hips and legs.
10. **Ekapaada prasaranaasana:** While inhaling, return to the position in step 4. Bring your left leg forward and place it between the hands. In the final pose, your right leg is stretched back, and the head is high.
11. **Uttanasana:** This is the same as the position in step 3. Exhale, and bring the right leg next to the left leg while raising the body. The head touches the knees.
12. **Back to namaskarasana:** As you inhale, raise the arms over your head and bend backwards in a repeat of step 2. After that, return to the position in step 1.

Note : *Do the exercise in a well-ventilated area, wearing minimal clothing. There are 12 positions in Surya Namaskar, and you should always go through the entire cycle. However, you can take some rest in between exercises. Ensure that your breathing is correct. Much of the benefit of Surya Namaskar is lost if you do not breathe in and out as recommended.*

Chapter 4

WALKING

Walking and running are natural, and very few would believe that there are right and wrong ways of walking and running. The difference is very marginal, however this would get multiplied if adopted as a means of exercise to keep fit. The rules are very elementary.

For a good aerobic workout, walk tall with your chest out and look straight directing all the motion forward. The arms should be bent at the waist level and not clenched into a tight fist, it should be loosely cupped. The movement of the arms should be to the side of the body, back and forth, and not side to side across the chest. The legs should move in two parallel lines. The body should be relaxed and the stride should be neither too long nor too short but just that comes naturally. No effort should be made to increase or decrease the stride.

Walking can be for different purpose, depending on the speed, purpose and technique. A stroll or leisure walking is slow walking, but at this level it can serve as useful exercise if done for a long time. Fitness walking is at a slightly faster speed and the body begins to sweat. Fitness walking should not be interrupted or halted but should be continuous. Hiking is walking for pleasure and sight seeing. Speed depends on the type of terrain, fitness levels and the weight being carried.

Walking can start any time, but not so with running. Jogging or slow running should be combined with walking to start with. Gradually the time devoted to walking should be gradually reduced. Cramps affect the body if one starts running after a long gap or without doing the warming up exercises. Cramps go away naturally as they come, and if they do not, they are a cause for concern and a doctor should be consulted. Most people take an upward jump while running, this has to change and a forward push is required to be taken.

Thought you mastered walking at age one? Well, think again. Fitness walking isn't an afternoon stroll. We're going to get all of you beginners moving with an easy walking programme that's guaranteed to help you get fit, toned, and on track with a fun cardiovascular workout.

Before you get started, let's run through some easy-to-follow walking tips. By following these key steps, you'll reduce your risk of injury; ensure that your body works at its peak.

Now you're ready to walk. This training programme will start you off and have you charging full-speed ahead in just seven weeks. Remember, take it slow, and be sensitive to your body. Don't push yourself on days when your tolerance is low, or if you feel the feet need to rest. Drink plenty of water, get lots of sleep, and don't forget to stretch after each walk to keep you in balance.

Walking Schedule

Week 1: This week hit the pavement for 10 minutes on three days. Watch your form as you walk.

Week 2: This week revv up your walking programme to 15 minutes on four days. Try the forward bend each day before you head out.

Week 3: This week log in 20 minutes of aerobic walking on four days. For maximum benefits, use a heart rate monitor and aim for your target heart rate (THR).

Week 4: Crank up your walking routine an extra notch, to 25 minutes and extend it to five days. Buy yourself a new pair of socks to celebrate.

Week 5: This week hold the line at five days, but add another five minutes to your programme. If you're feeling ambitious, work on your upper body on one of your free days.

Week 6: Maintain your five-day, 30-minute programme. Treat yourself to some soothing lotion. Massage your feet, using firm, circular motions, after your walk.

Week 7: Great going, now just keep walking.

Remember while Walking

1. **Stand up straight:** Look directly ahead. Imagine that a string is attached to the top of your head and is lifting you from the ground. Keep your shoulders back and relaxed, chest lifted, and tailbone pointing down to the ground.
2. **Relieve the stress points:** Relax your shoulders and shake out any tension from your arms and wrists. Bend your arms at the elbow about 83 degrees. Wiggle your fingers and then hold your hands in loose balls (pretend you're clasping a jumbo-size magic marker against your palms). Swing your arms naturally as you walk, but try not to let your hands extend above your chest.
3. **Keep your steps short and fast:** The faster you move, the better your cardiovascular workout. Keep an even stride and maintain a steady pace.
4. **Heel-to-toe motion:** As you walk, your heel should be the first part of your foot to hit the ground. Roll through the ball of the foot and push off with your toes. This motion reduces the risk of shin splints and tendon pulls.

Care of the Foot

1. **Blisters**: Blisters are caused when there is friction against the skin. Friction can be due to the friction between the ground and the foot (if not wearing any foot wear), and between the shoes and the skin. The shoes must fit properly when worn with the socks. Socks act as cushions, especially those made of cotton-acrylic. The socks should be clean and worn dry, on dry feet. Small blisters must be covered with sterile gauze pad. In case of a big blister, puncture it with a sterile needle and clean with antiseptic. Never peal off the skin over a blister.
2. **Calluses & corns:** These do not hurt, however, hard and big ones can be painful under pressure. Rubbing corns with pumice stone after a bath helps. A doctor can cut

or file the area. Applying body lotion can soften the area around a callus. Proper fitting shoes, corrected with pad or inserts can avoid callus and make running a pleasure.

3. **Bunions:** Bunions are painful swelling on the first joint of the big toe and these are usually hereditary. During walking or running they can get worse and very painful. Small swelling are generally overcome by wearing shoes that are wide in the front and with adequate cushioning. Surgery is recommended only if the bunion becomes painful.
4. **Nails:** Nail of the foot should be kept short and at no time should push against the front of the shoe. Nails rubbing against the shoe while running can be painful, the rubbing first occurs with the big toe. Care must be taken to cut the nails across so that they do not become ingrown.
5. **Athlete's foot:** It is a fungal growth on the feet. These occur when hygiene is lax and proper care is not taken of the feet. Shoes should be such that the foot is able to breathe. The shoes should be aired and kept in the sun if possible. Wear shoes dry and spray with anti fungal powder if the foot is affected. The area between the toes is most prone. In case of persistent problem consult a dermatologist.
6. **Cramps:** They are common problems. Simple cramps come and go easily. To avoid cramps, a little workout is necessary before any exercise. Massaging the feet after a workout helps to ease the muscles and prevent stiffness. If there is redness, swelling and pain, it is best to consult a doctor.

The bad news is that if your feet hurt, you're not going to enjoy your walk. The good news is that some common foot problems are fairly easy to treat and easier still to avoid.

Get rid of small irritants

To avoid blisters, stop them before they start. Keep your feet dry. Steer clear of cotton socks, which soak up perspiration and stretch out of shape. Wear socks made with fibres that draw moisture away from your skin. Or slip on a sock liner under your cotton socks. Rub petroleum jelly on your feet and between your toes before gearing up. This will reduce irritation that can lead to blisters. And finally, don't lace your shoes too tightly or too loosely. The pinching and rubbing may cause blister-forming irritation.

Precautions

- Pounding usually causes aching arches when you walk. The first thing you need to do is check your form. Are you landing on your heel and pushing off with your toes? If the problem persists, arch supports might help; if that doesn't work, consult a sports doctor.
- Corns and calluses are painful, and the more you ignore them, the worse they get. Check your shoes to make sure you've got a comfortable fit. And toss thin socks: You need to have a nice cushion between your feet and inside your shoes.
- Blackened toe nails are common and painful, and are caused when your big toe rubs against the front of your shoe. Keep your toe nails neatly trimmed and filed. Check your shoe size and wear double socks on the smaller foot if the shoe is too loose. Most people have one foot that's larger than the other. Always buy your walking shoes for the larger foot.

Two tension-relieving foot stretches

- Stand up straight, with your shoulders relaxed down. Hold your abdomien firmly to support your back and keep your pelvis in a neutral position (That's when your lower back has a natural curve but not too overarched). Your feet should be hip-wide apart. Place your hands on your waist. Slightly bend your knees. Shift your weight back onto your heels and lift your toes off the ground. Flex the front of your feet. Spread your toes as wide as you can. Hold the stretch for the count of five and don't forget to breathe. This will feel nice before you head out and later when you return home.

- Find a comfortable chair and practice picking up magic markers with your toes. Give your toes a nice press, grip the marker, lift your foot five to six inches off the ground, and then set it down. Do this exercise six times, alternating your feet.

Chapter 5

RUNNING

Don't despair, if you cannot run or have never run before, remember it's never too late for anything. Lack of motivation strikes even the most disciplined runners. Try to remember how good you felt about yourself after completing your last run and be proud that you've started a running programme at all.

Ten Tips to Keep Going

1. **Retail therapy:** New kicks may be just the jump-start you need. If your shoe soles look worn and the arch is drooping, it's time to shop. Most experts recommend at least one new pair a year. Remember, supportive, comfortable shoes are imperative to the health of your feet, ankles, and knees.
2. **Music motivation:** Try running with headphones. Make a tape of "get moving" songs or tune in to your favorite radio station. If you make a tape, record a few motivational quotes. Hearing your own voice will at least make you chuckle! Just be careful not to turn up the volume so high that you can't hear traffic!
3. **The early starter:** Some early birds find they are most likely to run first thing in the morning. Others have more energy in the evening. Try bringing running gear to work and trotting for lunch. Experiment to see what works best for you – or do a combination for variety.
4. **Routing out:** Break up the monotony by trying different routes – explore new areas in your town or drive to a park, beach, or new neighbourhood for a change of scenery.
5. **Speed limits:** Vary speed and intensity to stay focused and build endurance and strength. Mix running on flat ground with walking uphill, or try running fast for

20 seconds or longer and then jogging slowly to catch your breath.

6. **Get geared:** If you're not feeling motivated enough, just put on your running gear and aim for a ten-minute run. Once the shoes are on, you're less likely to back out. You may even surprise yourself once you get going and complete the entire run. If not, ten minutes is better than none!
7. **Find a buddy:** When someone else depends on us, we always perform better – or at least show up. Having someone to talk to while exercising can help pass the time, too.
8. **Set a goal:** Walks, race for a cause, or local fun runs are great events to keep you training, and they often have local clubs that will help you design a fitness plan. If you like to go solo, create your own goal: Run five miles, three hours, whatever you want. Just stick to it.
9. **Energize and zoom:** Keep up your energy by eating well (protein, carbohydrates, and fat included), taking rest days after long runs (at least one rest day a week), and staying hydrated throughout the day. Have healthy snacks before you run – junk food will slow you down.
10. **Put it in writing:** Make a running schedule and stick to it. Write down the days to run, how far to go, and which route to take. Once your schedule is in writing, you're more likely to do it. After your run, write down how it felt and what you thought of the route. Observe interesting landmarks. These schedules will mark your progress and help motivate you in the years to come.

Don'ts while Running

- ❑ Don't worry about the length of your stride, make it what come naturally and is comfortable.
- ❑ Don't lean too forward; keep the body straight and the head up.

- Don't run on your toes, try to land on the heel and roll the feet.
- Don't worry about the movement of the arms, move them naturally and bend them at the elbows.
- Don't run too fast for too long, or too much too early.

Chapter **6**

CYCLING

Indoor Cycling

This question is crucial. Despite its heavy promotion as a workout for even the most uncoordinated, indoor cycling is by no means for everyone. The intensity levels of many classes are far beyond what most novices or part-time exercisers can achieve and maintain, particularly for 40 minutes or more.

It's easy to get caught up in an instructor's chant of "Faster RPMs!" and "Don't sit down!" even if your body is telling you otherwise. That's why it's so important that participant either been in very good cardiovascular condition, or have the discipline to monitor and adhere to their body's cries for moderation.

Just because you may not be ready for a cycling class, now, doesn't mean you can't be in the very near future. Consider doing some cycle-specific training before you take your first indoor cycling class. Spend some time on a stationary bike, but make it interesting by creating your own "virtual" experience by "travelling" some of your favourite road trips in your mind as you listen to music. You can increase your endurance by interspersing periods of high-intensity cycling with more leisurely pedalling.

First Cycling Experience

- ❑ Don't make the mistake of showing up in your usual boxers or running shorts for cycling, there's no better way to make your ride unbearable. Opt instead for bike shorts, preferably padded like most outdoor cyclists wear. While this won't eliminate the chaffing and discomfort altogether, it helps a lot.
- ❑ Your second most important item is a full water bottle. Get ready to consume plenty of fluids during this class.

- Adjust the seat to the appropriate height. If the seat is too low, you won't be able to get enough leg extension on the down stroke. If it's too high, you'll be straining to reach and might injure yourself. Here's a good rule to follow: Your upstroke knee should never exceed hip level, while your down stroke knee should be about 85 percent straight. And don't grip the handlebars too tightly, as this will increase the tension in your neck and shoulders.
- Above all, concentrate on exercising at your own pace. Don't be intimidated by the high speeds and furious intensity of your cycling mates. Listen to your body and adjust the tension and speed accordingly, and don't be afraid to sit back and take a break when necessary.

Stationary Bikes Vs Moving bikes

The cheapest and most environment-friendly form of transportation, cycling doubles up as a very popular competitive sport as well. It provides an excellent cardiovascular exercise, which not only tones and strengthens the muscles but also provides a fun-filled escape from the four walls of a gym.

In the last decade or so, the only cycling most women have been doing has been on a stationary bike in the confines of a gymnasium. Many find it monotonous and boring. Fitness freaks swear by cycling which is more efficient than any other method of travelling, including walking. Nothing compares to cycling outdoors in the morning, inhaling the fresh air and absorbing the peace and quiet of the surroundings. Cycling around a garden or a green location induces relaxation while providing a workout as well. And while the stationary bike in a gym undoubtedly tones and strengthens the muscles, it can't quite provide the thrill of cycling rapidly down a lane and leaving the world behind!

Of course there are advantages to a stationary bike too. Biking indoors means no sudden rain, mud puddles or traffic to contend with. Using a stationary bicycle provides good alternative exercise and doesn't put excess strain on the hips, knees and feet. It's also the ideal solution for those who live in overcrowded metros with no space for cycling outdoors.

Acclimatise Body for Cycling

If you've decided to take up cycling for fitness, it will take some time for your body to adjust itself to the unexpected workout. You might find your thigh and calf muscles or arms becoming sore. There's nothing to worry about, though. After a few weeks, you'll get so used to it that you'll probably feel sore if you don't ride. Your legs provide the power for cycling. Your leg muscles attached to the thigh bone (femur) and the shin bone (tibia) will do the majority of the work. So if you have chubby legs or big hips, cycling is ideal for you. If you are tall, then your shins work out more; otherwise your thighbone usually works like a lever.

In the beginning, you may only be able to ride a few minutes. So keep it simple and without resistance in the beginning. You can increase resistance slightly every two weeks. If you are too fast in the beginning, your knees might hurt. This can make you stop too soon and will not benefit you. Keep your pedalling at a moderate speed. For most people, 50-60 revolutions per minute (rpm) is a good speed to start. As you get used to pedalling, you can increase your speed.

Cycling Tips

- Start with ten minutes a day and increase it gradually to twenty within ten to fifteen days. Half an hour of cycling at a comfortable speed, three to four times a week, is quite an ideal workout.
- Carry a towel and a water bottle when you venture out on your bike. Stop and drink a little water if you feel thirsty. If you get tired and out of breathe, slow down or rest before resuming. Keeping a record of the time will help you keep tabs on your progress.
- If you have your periods, you can try gentle cycling without any resistance.

- ❑ If you're riding a stationary bike, you can watch television, read, or listen to music to prevent boredom. You can even clip book holders to the handlebars to make reading easy.
- ❑ If you're taking up this activity, you might have to look after your diet as well. After all, you will not only be using different muscle groups but burning lots of calories as well. If you want to take cycling seriously, just remember that genetic inheritance, intensive training, and a competitive drive helps fitness freaks push the boundaries of endurance and speed on the bicycle.
- ❑ If you're planning to use your bike everyday, don't hesitate to buy a more expensive and durable model. This will work out cheaper in the long run since it hardly requires any maintenance. Do check if the bike suits your body type before blowing your cash. Buy from a good dealer who will give you at least a year's warranty.

Chapter 7

SWIMMING

Swimming is possibly one of the best exercises. It provides stamina, strength and suppleness. It is best suited for older people and people with back problems or arthritis. It is particularly good for people suffering from arthritis because there is no weight exerted on the joints, i.e., the hips and the knees. It is also a major aerobic exercise in which the major muscle groups are exercised with least risk of injury.

For swimming to have effect on the body, swimming must be continuous for minimum of 20 minutes. The most effective stroke is crawl. One should not swim long distances in the beginning, the distance should increase gradually. The most common effect of over exerting in the pool is sore shoulders. Perhaps the best part of swimming is that it is also a place where you can socialise and perhaps an exercise that can save your life.

Water contains chlorine and other additives, which can be harmful. The best way to protect the eyes and hair is to cover up, by wearing a water cap and goggles. Swimming can start at any age. You may adopt any stroke but what matters is how it is done. The strokes must be steady and continuous and in a rhythmic motion. In a crowded pool one must guard against colliding against one another, and if possible, peak timings must be avoided.

Swimming offers a low-impact, full-body workout. In addition, it's an ideal exercise for rehabilitating an injury. If you know how to swim the length of the pool, you can try this beginner swim programme. Keep in mind, it takes about 30 days to acclimate to swimming routine. Try doing this workout three times a week. If it feels too difficult, cut the distances in half. Build up by adding two lengths to the workout each week. Warm-up. Do 12 lengths (300 yards) of any stroke.

Swimming Programme

- ❑ Your warm-up should be no less than 10 minutes. Start by taking long, easy strokes and slowly build up the intensity, but not to a full speed. The idea is to stretch out, get a rhythm and start the blood flowing into the muscles.
- ❑ 4 lengths (100 yards) of freestyle are good enough. Repeat 3 times.
- ❑ Rest for a full minute between swims. Choose a speed that is challenging but consistent. 2 lengths (50 yards) kick. Repeat 4 times. Rest 45 seconds between each 2-length kick.
- ❑ Using a kickboard if you have one, alternate kicking on your back and stomach each length. If you don't have a kickboard, link your thumbs together with your arms above your head.
- ❑ On your stomach, kick with your face in the water, lifting your head to breathe.

Water Safety

- ❑ Do not go into the water alone.
- ❑ Do not swim in a place when there is no lifeguard on duty, unless you are a good swimmer.
- ❑ Do not swim if you are full, you may become nauseated in water. Children should be kept out of water for an hour after meals.
- ❑ Do not jump into the water if you cannot see the bottom, or if it is less than 9 feet deep.
- ❑ Do not drink alcohol before a swim. Non-alcoholic drinks are good.
- ❑ Do not enter open water in case of rain or approaching storm.
- ❑ Do not stay in cold water for long.

The Pilates Method of body conditioning promotes physical harmony and balance for people of all ages and physical conditions while providing a refreshing and energizing workout.

Diet and Action - The Fitness Combination

If you're overweight, eating your usual amount of calories while increasing activity is good for you, but eating fewer calories and being more active is even better. The following chart gives you an idea of the calories used per hour in common activities. Calories burned vary in proportion to body weight, however, so these figures are averages.

Activity - Calories Burned Per Hour

❑ Bicycling -	6 mph	240
❑ Bicycling -	12 mph	410
❑ Jogging -	5.5 mph	740
❑ Jogging -	7 mph	920
❑ Jumping rope	-	750
❑ Running in place	-	650
❑ Running -	10 mph	1,280
❑ Skiing (cross-country)	-	700
❑ Swimming -	25 yds/min	275
❑ Swimming -	50 yds/min	500
❑ Tennis (singles)	-	400
❑ Walking -	2 mph	240
❑ Walking -	4 mph	440

Calorie Burners

1. **Aerobics:** Aerobics is best. It used to be known as vigorous dancing and callisthenics set to invigorating music. But as fitness centres and classes have boomed over the years, and are full of innovative ideas, for a variety of workouts. The variety of classes available, have people flocking to the gym. Classes are popular because you have to keep up with an instructor who has already mapped out a variety of exercises to do at different times. Aerobics classes are particularly beneficial, because you're moving the entire time while

in class. They're great exercise for your legs, heart and lungs. (Depending on the type of aerobics you're into, you can burn about 250 calories in 30 minutes.)

2. **Jumping rope:** It is considered as a game amongst the young, but jumping rope is one of the most exhausting cardiovascular workouts you could ask for. Elite boxers use jumping rope as a conditioning tool. Contrary to popular belief, it is not just your legs that are getting the workout. In addition, your arms are moving the rope and if you're keeping good form, your body is tucking, moving and holding in muscles to end up with good tone. (Depending on your weight and the intensity of your jumping, you can burn about 300 calories in 30 minutes.)

3. **Kickboxing:** Combining moves from boxing with kicking moves one sees in martial arts, cardio kickboxing is a great workout for your heart, chest, arms, back and legs. People who do this type of exercise swear by its results, but it can take a while to burn higher numbers of calories because the moves are, for the most part, unfamiliar to new students. Take the time to learn proper form for all your moves. It will help you master the skills at a faster rate and burn calories more quickly. (Depending on your weight and the intensity of your workout, you can burn about 225 calories in 30 minutes.)

4. **Rock climbing:** During rock climbing, numerous muscles are engaged simultaneously as you carry your entire body weight up the rock face or climbing wall. Since you find yourself in numerous positions while on the wall, you're using muscles that otherwise get missed in traditional workouts. Be sure a certified instructor to guide you through the dangers and safety precautions before you start. Unlike more individual exercise programs, rock climbing is not a solitary pursuit. Some climbers feel that gyms are good training grounds, but the real climbing take place outdoors. It is always important to make sure you get help from an expert the

first time out. (Depending on your weight and activity intensity, you can burn about 320 calories in 30 minutes of rock climbing.)

5. **Tai chi:** Tai chi is similar to movements found in martial arts. The emphasis is on form and slow-flowing movements as you move from one position (form) to another. Tai Chi is a calculated, practiced, and designed to focus on the form; one needs to learn the proper techniques from the very beginning to reap the benefits of this great low-impact workout.

   Tai chi requires a good deal of concentration: You must learn to focus on specific muscles and how they relate to one another. Many of the poses demand strength, balance and some degree of coordination and thus involve your mind more than other cardiovascular activities. Another benefit of the slower pace is that many people feel calmed, not revved up by this activity. Though this is not an intensive workout as other activities, it is also a great exercise regimen for those recovering from injuries or illness, or older exercisers who are looking for a slower programme. (Depending on your weight and the intensity of your workout, you can burn about 120 calories in 30 minutes.)

6. **Rowing machine:** Rowing engages a number of muscles groups all at once and provides a great workout, even if you never hit the water. The most important thing to remember about rowing on an ergometer is your form. If you're unsure as to how to row or operate the machine, ask a trainer at your gym. If you use improper form, you can strain muscles.

   There are fun features on your ergometer that might inspire your next workout. Rowing is particularly good for your legs, arms, gluteus, back and abs. (Depending on your weight and the intensity of your workout, you can burn about 200 calories in 30 minutes.)

7. **Stair climber:** If you're out of breath at the top of a flight of stairs, the last thing you might want to look into at

the gym is a stair-climbing machine, right? Actually, stair climbers continue to be some of the most popular machines at the gym. In particular, they target your legs and glutes and help you break into a sweat faster than a lot of machines. (Depending on your weight and the intensity of your workout, you can burn about 180 calories in 30 minutes.)

8. **Treadmill running:** Treadmills are a long-time favourite of gym-goers everywhere. Indoor running on a treadmill has a number of advantages: It allows you to train even in bad weather, it provides you with a gentler running surface than asphalt and it keeps you near all the other equipment at the end of your run. Most treadmills are equipped with mechanisms that allow you to alter the incline of the track, as well as the speed at which you want to run. (Depending on your weight and the intensity of your workout, you can burn about 370 calories in 30 minutes.)

9. **Racquet sports:** Whether you play tennis, racquetball, squash or other racquet sports, you're sure to get a good cardio workout, as well as improve your coordination and gain some agility. Racquet sports involve a lot of start-and-stop play, so be prepared to burn fewer calories than when you engage in activities that offer continuous movement. But the bonus of racquet sports is that you play them against a competitor, and with that comes a natural fighting spirit that you wouldn't necessarily have on a treadmill. The whole idea of racquet sports is that they're fun to play. The bonus is you get beneficial exercise. (Depending on your weight and the intensity of the workouts, you can burn about 240 calories in 30 minutes.)

10. **Golf:** Though it's known as a leisure sport, golf still qualifies as cardiovascular exercise, especially if you carry your own clubs and don't use the golf cart. Remember: You should get 30 minutes of exercise three to four times weekly but it doesn't have to be continuous.

It's okay to grab 10 minutes here and there, which is why golf is still good for you. (Depending on your weight, how much you walk and equipment you carry, you can burn about 170 calories in 30 minutes.)

11. **Swimming:** Swimming is a great way of burning the extra calories because it is pleasurable. Depending on you weight and the intensity of your swim, you can burn about 240 calories in 30 minutes.
12. **Yoga:** Depending on you weight and the intensity and type of yoga practiced, you can burn about 120 calories in 30 minutes.
13. **Cycling:** Depending on you weight and the intensity and distance of your ride, you can burn about 240 calories in 30 minutes.
14. **Walking:** Depending on you weight and the intensity and distance of your fitness walk, you can burn about 140 calories in 30 minutes.
15. **Running:** Depending on you weight and the intensity and distance of your run, you can burn about 340 calories in 30 minutes.

Chapter 8

EXERCISING EQUIPMENTS

Begin your fitness programme by getting to know what technique you should be using for the equipment or activity you are doing. Putting the emphasis on technique first will pay off long-term with not only better results but lower your risk of injury. Don't try to change your body in a few weeks or even in a couple of months. This is the body you've spent years creating or destroying. Take a long-term approach to changing or rebuilding it.

Endurance Equipment

Endurance routines can be done with aerobic or strength equipment. The fundamental concept is to gently work a muscle or group of muscles much more thoroughly. This must be done only after a conditioning period that you build up to over a period of time. If you suddenly work a muscle to exhaustion without this preparation, you are sure to get injured. Pieces of equipment that naturally lend them to this concept of working out more thoroughly with a minimum of risk of injury are, rowers and steppers.

Don't forget the all reliable dumbbells and wrist ankle weights. An aerobic warm-up involving that part of your body is necessary before you do endurance segments of your fitness routine. This ensures that you have warmed-up and stretched the muscles to be worked out. It also enhances the muscle's ability to remove waste products such as lactic acid more effectively so you can do as much of that routine prior to fatigue.

Aerobic Equipment

Most people have heard how important it is to get your heart working out for general health. This is a fact, if you are not engaging in activities that raise your heart rate for sustained periods. Aerobic workouts mean activities working with oxygen. Than means getting muscles working actively enough that they require large amounts of oxygen to do their work. Naturally, your heart gets the oxygen from your lungs and pumps it through your body. One of the many benefits of most aerobic activities is the muscle fitness, joint fitness, and of course, the exhilarating and relaxing benefits of working out. Aerobic equipment includes treadmills (which are probably the easiest to do since it is the most natural), all styles of upright and recumbent exercise bikes, since it works both the arms and legs. Other good aerobic categories include rowers, slide boards and steppers.

While Buying equipment

1. **Don't overbuy features:** Like moths to a flame, people are drawn to cardiovascular equipment that has every conceivable readout and calculation. These gadgets often go unused, though, so they may not be the best place to spend your money.
2. **Don't skimp on the basics:** Sturdy construction and smooth, quiet operation are what matter most. For example, with treadmills, good deck cushioning and stability are key factors to look for.
3. **Avoid fast or sight-unseen purchasing:** Almost any treadmill works fine during the first few minutes. Only when doing a longer workout will you notice things like excessive vibration and noise. For cardio machines, spend at least 20 minutes trying different programmes, for strength equipment, do a set of 10 repetitions.
4. **Don't ignore the top of the line:** If you don't try the best equipment first, you won't know what quality features to look for. Stay away from infomercial products or other low-price equipment. A store specializing in fitness equipment is probably the best place to start your search. It's not a bad idea to stick to brands you've used at health clubs - a manufacturer's quality often carries over into home models.

5. **Don't overestimate your abilities:** An exercise or movement that looks easy on TV may not work for you. For example, some machines may offer an outstanding cardio workout, but they also require a high level of concentration and coordination. When purchasing a strength-training machine, look for one with simple procedures for changing weights. If adjusting the weight isn't mind-numbingly simple, you're likely not to do it!
6. **Don't limit your options:** Although treadmills are extremely popular and reliable, elliptical trainers also provide functional movement with lots of variety. Stationary bikes - both upright and recumbent are very popular. Stair steppers, rowing machines, home gyms and equipment for home-based exercise have a large variety.
7. **Don't ignore your personal comfort:** Make sure the rowing machine you are thinking of buying doesn't put too many demands on your back. If you are looking at treadmills and are overweight or have orthopaedic concerns, check for sturdy handrails, gradual pace changes and structural integrity. Look for a home gym that will adjust to your body height and size.
8. **Don't believe everything you hear:** Some fitness products that sound great on infomercials have limited effectiveness. Abdominal exercise devices, for example, don't really offer any results beyond those achieved by doing abdominal exercises without equipment.
9. **Don't go it alone:** Ask questions of other exercisers and fitness professionals, as well as equipment representatives. Before buying, find out about equipment delivery, set-up, and warranties and return policies.

5 Point Exercise Programme

1. Warm Up (5 minutes)
2. Aerobic Exercise (20 - 25 minutes)
3. Strength Training (10 - 20 minutes)
4. Flexibility and Relaxation Exercises (10 - 15 minutes)
5. Cool down (10 minutes)

Warming Up

1. Stand with your feet a shoulder-width apart, your arms at your sides. Gently roll your head in a half circle in front of you, back and forth a few times. With your head straight, drop your left ear to your shoulder and hold. Bring your head to centre and drop your right ear to your shoulder and hold. Bring your head back up and drop your chin to your chest. Head up and drop it back. Bring your head back up and face forward.
2. Shrug your shoulders up and release; repeat this six times. Roll your shoulders backward six times; roll them forward six times.
3. Place your left hand on your hip and raise your right arm up. Keeping your torso straight, reach your right arm over your head, bending to the left from your waist. Hold and then return to the normal position. Repeat with the left arm reaching over your head to the right. You should feel a stretch in your sides.
4. Stand with your feet slightly more than a shoulder-width apart. Reach down your left leg as far as you can, trying to touch your ankle or toes if possible. Hold for ten seconds. Slowly roll yourself upright, keeping your head down to avoid dizziness. Now reach down your right leg in the same manner and hold. Again, roll up slowly with your head down. This stretches the muscles at the back of your leg.
5. Still standing with your feet apart, turn to your left. Bend your left knee and extend your right leg straight out behind you. Centre your body so that your left knee is bent at a 90-degree angle to the floor. Hold this position, called a runner's stretch, for a count of ten, gently pressing your straight leg down toward the floor. You'll feel the stretch in the thigh muscle of the out- stretched leg. Repeat this exercise with your right leg.
6. To stretch your Achilles tendon and calf muscles, stand two to three feet from a wall and place your hands on it. Keeping your legs straight and your feet flat on the floor, lean in to the wall. You should feel the stretch in

your legs; hold it for ten seconds. Try stepping back a bit farther to increase the stretch; remember that your feet should remain flat on the floor.

Exercising and Conditioning

With all of the following exercises, be sure to do the repetitions slowly and evenly, with some tension in your limbs. Your arms should not simply swing back and forth, but should move in a controlled, deliberate way, almost as if they were resisting against an invisible weight.

All of these suggest ten repetitions, but if you are just starting out, do as many as you feel comfortable doing. "No pain, no gain" may be true to some extent for accomplished athletes, but for the average person, pain often signifies stress. Try to stay tuned to the sensations in your muscles and use common sense. If it hurts too much, it's time to stop. As you exercise, your muscle tissue actually breaks down. In order to allow your muscles time to restore them, work out every other day or exercise various body areas on alternating days.

Arms

1. Stand with your feet a shoulder-width apart, stomach tucked in, and back straight. Extend your arms out to the sides with your palms facing out. Bring your arms in together straight out in front of you with the palms inwards. Now extend the arms backwards, stretching them out as far as possible, palms facing each other. Do ten repetitions.
2. Keeping your arms extended, bring them straight up together above your head, and then drop them so that they extend out to the sides. Repeat ten times.
3. Arms still extended with palms facing out, move your arms forward in small circles. Do ten of these and then increase to a medium-size circle. Do ten repetitions and then ten more, making the largest circle you can. Repeat this cycle, moving your arms backward.
4. Extend your arms out to the sides, bend them at the elbows, and make fists. Squeeze your bent arms together

so that your forearms meet in front of you. This exercise works the chest and arms.

5. To work your biceps, extend your arms straight down at your sides with your inner forearms and fists facing up. Bending at the elbow, squeeze your fists to your shoulders. In order to obtain the maximum benefit, pretend that there is a weight on your inner forearm and resist against the pressure as you squeeze up.

Waist

1. Standing with your feet a shoulder-width apart, bend to the left, reaching slightly down and out as far as you can with your left arm. Your right hand can remain on your hip or your elbow can rise up simultaneously as you are reaching to the side with your left arm. Do ten repetitions and then repeat with the right side.
2. Standing with your feet apart, place your hands on your hips or raise your arms to chest level and bend them at the elbows so that your forearms are directly in front of your chest. Keeping your hips straight, move from the waist, twisting ten times to the left and ten times to the right. Then try alternating, pausing in the forward position, between each twist.
3. This one may be a little harder to do. Sit on the floor with your legs spread open as wide as possible and your hands clasped behind your head. Keeping your back straight and your elbows back, reach down toward the floor behind your left knee with your left elbow. Come up, pause, and then reach down toward the floor with your right elbow. Do ten repetitions.

Abdomen

1. Sit on the floor with your knees slightly bent and your back straight. You can hold your arms straight out in front of you for balance, or you can cross them over your chest. From this sitting position, slowly roll back so that your shoulders are just a few inches above the floor. Pause and then slowly roll back up to a sitting po-

sition. As you do this exercise, always press the small of your back downward, rather than arching your back, in order to prevent strain. Do ten repetitions.

2. Lie on the floor with your stomach tucked in so that the small of your back presses down toward the floor. Bend your knees slightly and keep your feet flat on the floor. Clasp your hands behind your head, and, keeping your elbows back as much as possible, slowly raise your head and shoulders up off the ground. In order to help you do this exercise properly, pick a spot on the ceiling and raise your chin up toward that spot. Your head, neck, and shoulders should stay aligned and straight; you should not be "hunching" up, tucking your chin in, or using your elbows and arms to pull you up. If you don't do this exercise in the proper way, your abdomen will not benefit at all. If you do it properly, however, you will feel your abdominal muscles contract as you come up and relax as you come down. Do ten repetitions slowly and rhythmically.
3. This is a more advanced form of exercise 2. Lying in the same position, rest your left leg on your right knee. Lift your head and shoulders up in the same manner as above. Do ten repetitions and then switch legs for ten more.

Thighs

Sit on the floor with your back straight, your hands on the floor to your sides and slightly behind you with your arms straight to support your body. Keeping your right leg relaxed, straighten your left leg, point your toe, and slowly raise it up about a foot off the ground. Lower the leg and repeat ten times. Switch legs and repeat ten times with your right leg. Remember to keep your back straight as you do this exercise.

Inner Thighs

Sitting in the same position as in the "Thighs" exercise with your legs extended straight out in front of you, lift your left leg a few inches off the floor, point your toe, and slowly move it out to the left. You'll feel a nice stretch on the inside of your thigh. Bring your leg back to the starting position, and repeat ten times. Switch legs and repeat ten times with your right leg.

Outer Thighs

Lie on your left side, your left arm bent at the elbow so that your hand supports your head, your legs stacked on top of each other. Make sure that your back is straight, and tilt your pelvis slightly toward the floor. Bend your bottom leg at the knee and keep this leg relaxed. Straighten your top leg, toe pointed, and raise it up as far as you can. You want to keep your leg straight as you raise it so that the outer thigh is parallel with the ceiling. Lower your leg and repeat ten times. When you do this exercise, pretend that there is a weight on your outer thigh and resist against it as you raise your leg. This will maximize the benefit to your muscles. Do ten repetitions and then lie on your opposite side and work your opposite leg.

Buttocks

Lie on your back, your knees bent with your feet apart, your hands clasped behind your head or placed under your buttocks. Without arching your back, lift your buttocks off the floor. Squeeze your buttocks with each lift and then release as you come back to the floor. Do ten repetitions with your feet apart and then ten with your feet together. As you master this exercise, you can do it keeping your feet apart with your knees together; with your feet together and your knees spread apart. Those who are more advanced can cross one leg over the opposite knee and vice versa.

Using the stretches described in the warm-up, be sure to spend at least five minutes cooling down after your exercise routine. If you do aerobic exercise, cool down by slowing your pace for five minutes as well as doing five minutes of stretching exercises. For example, when you're done jogging or bicycling, take a brisk walk to cool down; if you swim, cool down by doing gentle breast-, back-, or sidestrokes for five minutes. Although you may be tempted sometimes to skip the stretching, remember that your muscles have contracted and tightened during exercise, and they must be stretched out in order to prevent cramping and injuries, such as pulls.

Tips to Make Exercise a Habit

- ❑ Choose an activity you enjoy.
- ❑ Tailor your programme to your own fitness level.
- ❑ Set realistic goals.
- ❑ Choose an exercise that fits your lifestyle.
- ❑ Give your body a chance to adjust to your new routine.
- ❑ Don't get discouraged if you don't see immediate results.
- ❑ Don't give up if you miss a day; just get back on track the next day.
- ❑ Find a partner for a little motivation and socialization.
- ❑ Build some rest days into your exercise schedule.
- ❑ Listen to your body. If you have difficulty breathing or experience faintness or prolonged weakness during or after exercise, consult your physician.

It's a good idea to choose more than one type of exercise to give your body a thorough workout and to prevent boredom. Also, you might want to choose one indoor exercise and one outdoor activity to allow for changes in your schedule or for inclement weather. Very few people live in a climate that's temperate year-round. But weather extremes don't have to interfere with your exercise routine if you make some minor adjustments.

When it's Hot or Humid

- ❑ Exercise during cooler and/or less humid times of day. Try early morning or evening. Drink plenty of fluids, especially water. Avoid alcohol, which encourages dehydration. Wear light, loose-fitting clothing.
- ❑ Stop at the first sign of muscle cramping or dizziness.

When it's Cold

- ❑ Dress in layers.
- ❑ Wear gloves or mittens to protect your hands.

- ❑ Wear a hat or cap. Up to 40% of body heat is lost through your neck and head.
- ❑ Adjust the size of your shoes if you need to wear thicker socks.
- ❑ Warm up slowly.
- ❑ Drink plenty of fluids. You can get dehydrated in the winter also.
- ❑ Stop if you experience shivering, drowsiness or disorientation.

Year-round Safety

- ❑ Let someone know where you're going and when you'll be back.
- ❑ Carry identification with you when exercising outside the home.
- ❑ Build in warm-up and cool-down periods to decrease risk of injury.
- ❑ Avoid strenuous exercise for one to two hours after eating.
- ❑ Wear sturdy, well-fitting shoes appropriate for the activity.
- ❑ Wear brightly coloured clothing when exercising outdoors.
- ❑ Add lights and reflector tape to your body or bike if you exercise after dark.
- ❑ Wear helmets and safety pads appropriate for the activity.
- ❑ Move against traffic if you must run or walk on the road.
- ❑ Don't let headphones distract you from observing traffic and safety concerns.
- ❑ Avoid heavily polluted areas and exercise indoors if you have heart or lung disease. Avoid areas where traffic is heavy.
- ❑ Take special care of your feet if you are diabetic or have vascular disease.

Checking Health

If you're under 35 and in good health, you don't need to see a doctor before beginning an exercise programme. But if you are over 35 and have been inactive for several years, you should consult your physician, who may or may not recommend a graded exercise test. Other conditions that indicate a need for medical clearance are - high blood pressure, heart trouble, family history of early stroke or heart attack deaths, frequent dizzy spells, extreme breathlessness after mild exertion, arthritis or other bone problems, severe muscular and ligament or tendon problems. Vigorous exercise involves minimal health risks for persons in good health or those following a doctor's advice. Far greater risks are present by habitual inactivity and obesity.

Buddy support – This is sometimes the hardest part to co-ordinate since so many people have different schedules. For those of us who need a support system, call a couple of friends and tell them that this is something important to you and that you'd like them to keep checking up on you to see that you are on track

Having a definite schedule and someone counting on you can make the workouts in between easier to get through. If you and a friend have two or more pieces of fitness equipment at your homes, alternate whose house the workout is at. Make it a round robin with a few friends. Fun runs, bike-a-thons, and more can be made more fun when you get friends involved. After all, life is not just about us, it is about getting out and being with other people we care about. Maybe you need to be the one who's checking-up on someone who needs that support. And by the way, be creative and have fun!

Stop Making Excuses

You can probably come up with plenty of excuses for why you're not more active. You're too young, you're too old, you're too busy, you're too tired or you're in pretty good shape - for your age. But with few exceptions, these excuses are pretty flimsy. There are activities for the young and old and for those with little time. So the next time you think about getting fit, don't ask, "Who has time?" Instead, ask yourself "Who doesn't want to feel better?"

SECTION 2

SLIMMING

Chapter 9

OBESITY

Thanks to all the hype generated by the beauty contests and advertisements, one message that has gone across is that 'slim is beautiful'. This has led to a growing awareness about diet and weight loss. On the flip side, it has also generated a host of unhealthy fad diets, which promise to melt away the fat without any pain.

Obesity is becoming the single leading cause for many ailments. Right from high blood pressure to diabetes, it is the root cause of all problems. The changing lifestyle has led to the birth of a generation that is increasingly becoming unhealthy. Lack of exercise, fast food and stress, all have added to the growing number of obese people in the society. In this age of computers when the only kind of exercise is the moving of a mouse, fat is not burnt but accumulated in the body. This accumulated fat results into an obese condition.

In a way it is good that weight loss has become an obsession with most people because being overweight means to invite a whole lot of diseases. Obesity is defined simply as an excess of body fat. Your body is made up of water, fat, protein, carbohydrate and various vitamins and minerals. It is the excess fat that causes the problems.

Causes of obesity

1. **Obesity and hypertension:** It has been proved beyond any doubt that hypertension is a common outcome of obesity. In overweight young adults, age 20-45, the prevalence of hypertension is 6 times that of their normal-weight peers. We all know that fat children, generally, make fat adults and weight gain in young adult life is a potent risk factor for the later development of hypertension. In races where people tend to weigh

less with advancing years, cases of hypertension are infrequent. Doctors have also found that the distribution of fat in the body may have an important affect on blood pressure risk. People with more flab and fat in the abdomen or upper body region are more likely to suffer from high blood pressure than those with lower body fat in the gluteal or thigh region. In obese persons, an accumulation of abdominal fat results in the release of free fatty acids into the portal vein, which causes incidents of insulin resistance and hyperinsulinemia.

2. **Obesity and diabetes:** Even moderate obesity, particularly abdominal obesity, can increase the risk of non-insulin dependent diabetes mellitus (NIDDM), ten-fold. Fat tissue apparently has two roles in promoting diabetes: it increases the demand for insulin and, in obese individuals; it creates insulin resistance, and, therefore, hyperinsulinemia. It is possible that nutrients are preferably sent into fat for storage. Some of the insulin resistance in obesity can be attributed to a decrease in insulin receptors. Weight reduction in the obese NIDDM can lead to improvement of glycemic control as well as improvement of related medical problems such as hypertension or hyperlipidemia.

3. **Obesity - cardiovascular disease and fat distribution:** In recent findings, an increased risk of cardiovascular disease has been noted with increasing obesity. In a recent finding doctors calculated that, for each 10% increase in body weight in men, there is approximately a 20% increase in the incidence of coronary artery disease. For every 10% increase in relative body weight, the following effects take place:

   - ❑ Systolic blood pressure increases 6.5 mm/Hg,
   - ❑ Plasma cholesterol 12 mg/dL and
   - ❑ Fasting blood glucose 2 mg / dL.

   Most men tend to accumulate fat in the midriff region and both the degree of obesity and the distribution of body fat, independently and collectively contribute to the risk factors for cardiovascular disease. The simplest way to measure the degree of abdominal obesity is to record the waist circumference and divide it by the hip circumference. In men, the risk of cardiovascular disease increases sharply when waist/hip ratio (WHR) is above 1.0. In women the same disease risks increase when the WHR is above 0.8. Numerous reports have indicated that a high proportion of abdominal fat is associated with insulin resistance, hyperinsulinemia, impaired glucose tolerance, diabetes, and an elevated blood pressure.

To assess cardiovascular risk, the Waist-Hip ratio should be used simultaneously with total body fat.

4. **Obesity and cancer:** Overweight men have a significantly higher mortality rate for colorectal and prostate cancer; men whose weight is 130% or more above average are 2.5 times more likely to die of prostate cancer during a 20 year follow-up, compared to men of average weight. Women, who have gone through their menopause and have upper body fat accumulation, have an increased risk of developing breast cancer. Overweight women also have higher rates of cancer of uterus and ovaries.

5. **Obesity and endocrine abnormalities:** Obese women, especially those with upper body obesity, show more irregularity in menstrual cycles as well as greater frequency of other menstrual abnormalities than normal weight women. They also have more problems during pregnancy with an increased frequency of toxaemia and hypertension. In obese girls, the onset of menarche occurs at a younger age than in normal weight girls. This could be due to the fact that menstruation is probably initiated when body weight reaches a critical mass.

6. **Obesity and gall bladder:** Obese women in the 20-30 year age range have a six-fold increase in the risk of developing gall bladder disease compared to normal-weight women. By age 60, nearly one-third of obese women can be expected to have developed gall bladder disease.

For each kilogram of fat, approximately 20 mg/dL of cholesterol is synthesized. In obese persons, the bile is therefore more saturated with cholesterol. Likewise, fatty infiltration of the liver is associated with obesity.

7. **Obesity and pulmonary abnormalities:** There are several abnormalities in pulmonary function in obese individuals. As an individual becomes more obese, the muscular work required for respiration increases. In addition, respiratory muscles may not function normally in obese individuals.
8. **Obesity and arthritis:** It has also been found that incidence of arthritis is higher in obese people. Although the cause is unclear, there is a significant correlation between uric acid levels, which causes arthritis, and weight. In the 45-64 year old age group, the prevalence of gout goes up dramatically when relative weight is higher by 130%, above desirable. An increase in body weight adds pressure to weight bearing joints. In middle-aged women excess body weight is a major reason for the osteoarthritis of the knee. The good news is that losing weight can, markedly, decrease the chance of developing osteoarthritis.
9. **Obesity and functional and psychological disorders:** The obese individuals are slower, more lethargic and inactive. This affects their activities of daily living. Obese patients also have physical incapacity due to back and joint problems and shortness of breath. This contributes to their proneness to fatal accidents and falls.

Research proves that in the severely obese people, there is an increased incidence of absenteeism and unemployment. Discrimination against obese persons is common in both academic and work settings. This leads to significant erosion in their body image, which is the major form of psychological disturbance specific to obese persons. Emotional disturbances are often likely to be a consequence of obesity rather than the cause. However, in some studies, obese persons were found to be significantly less anxious and depressed than normal weight persons.

How Fat Accumulates?

Accumulation of fat is the result of eating more food than the body needs for its daily expenditure of energy. Thus fat represents the body's main reserve of available energy. The body of a healthy 20-year-old man is about 20% fat. This rises to 25% by the time he is 50. The softer bodies of women contain a correspondingly greater proportion of fat. A 20-year-old girl's body is 25% fat. This rises to 45% by the time she is 50. Not only do women have a thicker layer of fat under the skin than men, it tends to be concentrated around certain areas, notably the breasts, buttocks and legs.

The table given here demonstrates the distribution of fat pads in the various parts of the body.

Fat Pad	Man	Woman
Shoulder	18	18
Outside arm	4	6
Inside arm	4	7
Hip	19	19
Top of thigh	16	28
Outside leg	5	7
Inside leg	6	11
Front of the leg	3	4
Back of the leg	7	13

Body composition

The body of a healthy individual is composed as –

Water – 60% (intracellular & extracellular)
Fat – 18%
Protein – 16%
Carbohydrates – 0.7%
Minerals – 5.2%
Fat is distributed in the following manner-
Subcutaneous tissue – 50%
In abdominal cavity – 10-15%
In renal space – 10-15%
Intra-muscular space – 5%

Is fat necessary?

Fat is required for cushioning joints and organs, protection of organs, regulation of body temperature and storing vitamin. So, we can't eliminate it totally from our diet. But, it definitely needs to be controlled to the desirable level.

Energy requirement

Most of us understand that weight management depends upon the energy balance equation; the amount of energy you put into your body (food calories) versus the amount of energy you expend (activity). It is logical that a person consuming more calories, than is required by his body for the daily activities, is likely to store the extra calories as fat. But how do you know how many calories your body needs to reach or maintain a certain weight?

Understanding your body's energy requirements can help guide you when making nutritional choices. We'll show you two ways to determine your energy requirements, the accurate way and the easy way.

The Accurate Way

There are three primary components that make up your body's energy expenditure. Adding these three components together, basal metabolic rate, energy expended during physical activity, and the thermic effect of food is the most accurate way of determining how many calories your body requires each day.

Basal metabolic rate (BMR) – Most of the body's energy, about 60-70%, goes to supporting the ongoing metabolic work of the body's cells. This includes such activities as heart beat, respiration and maintaining body temperature. Here is a simple method to determine your BMR:

For adult males – Multiply the body weight by 10; add double the body weight to this value. [i.e., for a 150 lb male, 1,500 + (2 x 150)=1,800 cal/day BMR]

For adult females – Multiply body weight by 10; add the body weight to this value. [i.e., for a 120 lb female, 1,200 + 120=1,320 cal/day BMR]

Energy expended during physical activity - The second component of the equation depends upon your level of physical activity. Physical activity has a profound effect on human energy expenditure and contributes 20-30% to the body's total energy output. One of the most reliable methods in calculating calories burned during physical activity is the Metabolic Energy (MET) Method.

Thermic effect of food - The last component to calculate has to do with your body's management of food. The increase in energy required to digest food is referred to as the thermic effect of food (TEF) and it's simple to determine:

TEF = total kcals consumed x 10% [i.e., 2,000 kcals consumed/day x 0.10 = 200 kcals expended for TEF]

The Easy Way

If all of those calculations seem too confusing or tedious, you can roughly estimate your daily calorie requirements using this simple formula:

For sedentary people:

Weight x 14 = estimated cal/day

For moderately active people:

Weight x 17 = estimated cal/day

For active people:

Weight x 20 = estimated cal/day

*(**Note:** Moderately Active is defined as 3-4 aerobic sessions per week. Active is defined as 5-7 aerobic sessions per week).*

Body Composition and its importance

The waist circumference and the body mass index (B.M.I.) are indirect methods to assess a person's body composition. The waist-to-hip ratio (W.H.R.) is another index of body fat distribution. However, WHR is less accurate than waist circumference and is no longer a recommended measure. What is the waist circumference?

The waist circumference is a simple measure around a person's natural waist (just above the navel). A high-risk waistline is defined as more than 35 inches (88 cm) for women, and more than 40 inches (102 cm) for men.

What is Body Mass Index (BMI)?

The body mass index is a formula to assess a person's body weight relative to height. It's a useful, indirect measure of body composition, because it co-relates highly with body fat in most people. Weight in kilograms is divided by height in meters squared (kg/m2). Or multiply weight in pounds by 705, divide by height in inches, then divide again by height in inches.

How to find Body Mass Index?

- Use a weighing scale on a hard, flat, uncarpeted surface. Wear very little clothing and no shoes.
- Obtain your weight to the nearest kilogram and write it down. With your eyes facing forward and your heels together, stand very straight against a wall. Your buttocks, shoulders and the back of your head should be touching the wall.

Use a ruler held at a right angle to the wall to mark your height at the highest point of your head. Then use a yardstick held flat against the wall to measure from the floor to the point you marked with the ruler. Write down your height in metres to the nearest centimetre.

For example – if your height is 1.65 metres and weight is 59 kgs.

$$\text{BMI} = \frac{\text{Weight (kg)}}{\{\text{Height (m)}\}^2}$$

$$= \frac{59}{(1.65)^2}$$

$$= 21.7$$

Some people who have trained bodies with dense muscle mass may have a high BMI score but very little body fat. For them the waist circumference, the skin-fold or fat-fold measurements, or more direct methods of measuring body fat may be more useful.

Body Mass Index (for adults)

	Females	Males
Acceptable BMI	19-24	20-25
Moderately High BMI	25-30	26-30
Very High BMI	30+	30+

Height	Minimal risk (BMI under 25)	Moderate risk (BMI 25-29.9)	Overweight High risk (BMI above 30)
4'10"	118 lbs. or less	119-142 lbs.	143 lbs. or more
4'11"	123 or less	124-147	148 or more
5'0	127 or less	128-152	153 or more
5'1"	131 or less	132-157	158 or more
5'2'	135 or less	136-163	164 or more
5'3"	140 or less	141-168	169 or more
5'4"	144 or less	145-173	174 or more
5'5"	149 or less	150-179	180 or more
5'6"	154 or less	155-185	186 or more
5'7"	158 or less	159-190	191 or more
5'8"	163 or less	164-196	197 or more
5'9"	168 or less	169-202	203 or more
5'10"	173 or less	174-208	209 or more
5'11"	178 or less	179-214	215 or more
6'0"	183 or less	184-220	221 or more
6'1"	188 or less	189-226	227 or more
6'2"	193 or less	194-232	233 or more
6'3"	199 or less	200-239	240 or more
6'4"	204 or less	205-245	246 or more

(Note – 1 pound=0.454 kg)

Once you have discovered that you are over-weight, the next step is to lose weight through proper diet and exercise regimen.

Chapter 10

HOW TO LOSE EXTRA WEIGHT?

The key to losing weight is dependent on just two factors – **Eating behaviour** and **Effective Exercise**.

Most people who are overweight make a serious attempt at some point or the other. Many do not succeed or, if they do, put the weight on again within a few weeks or months. Why does this happen? The reason is that most slimmers see the measures they are taking to lose weight as temporary. They are not actually attempting to change their basic lifestyle, so the weight loss does not become permanent. Slimmers cannot be blamed for this. In the past it has been assumed that it was only necessary for someone to be given the correct information about the calorie values of foods and what target to aim for, and then they could lose weight. Failure was considered to be due to lack of will power.

Eating Behaviour

Eating behaviour is nothing but – How you eat, what you eat and how much you eat.

Controlling the food factor

Now, we know that many factors influence a person's eating habits and that if a person is to lose weight successfully then he or she must first identify these factors and learn to control them. The reason most people fail to slim is that the factors, which decide their weight, have got beyond their control. It is essential to take steps to bring them back within control. Overeating has been proved to be caused as much by the situation surrounding a person as by the person himself. If a situation can be controlled then overeating can be brought under control too. The first step to take is to analyse the situation and discover the factors, which affect your eating.

The way to do this is to keep a daily eating record. Every time you eat you should record –

- ❑ What the food is.
- ❑ The food you ate.
- ❑ How much food you ate.
- ❑ Where you were.
- ❑ What you were doing.
- ❑ Who you were with.
- ❑ What feeling you had while you ate.

After keeping an eating record for a few days, you will begin to see patterns in your eating habits. For example, you may see that you ate a lot when you were by yourself and you felt lonely, or that you ate a lot of problem foods such as chocolates, biscuits or peanuts. Alternatively, it may be that you eat most in company and so you should seek ways of altering your social habits. You might arrange to meet a friend in a sports club rather than in a café or pub.

Strategies for losing weight

To lose weight, one has to put in a determined and genuine effort. It is not an easy task nor is it a quick one. The efforts may not lead to visible effect, immediately. In fact, a lot many people give up too soon or make a half-hearted effort. Here are some useful guidelines for those who, really, want to lose the flab.

How to control eating habits?

You can begin to control your eating by developing a series of rules, which you undertake to use for guidance. Occasionally, you may break a rule. That does not mean that you have failed, just start again. First, you must learn to control all the circumstances that precede eating, then eating itself. Then the consequence of eating – your weight – will come under your control.

Choose a particular room in which to eat at home and only eat there

If you choose to eat in the kitchen, then it means you must not eat in the living room even if you want to watch TV. If you want to watch, eat later. If you choose to eat in the living room, then you must not nibble while you are in the kitchen. Make up your mind to eat in only one place in the room, and when you eat avoid doing other things at the same time such as watching TV or listening to music. In this way, you will gradually reduce the number of situations, which make you think of food. If you are in the habit of eating while watching TV, then switching on the set becomes a cue for the conditioned reaction of eating. In the same way, being in a particular room such as the kitchen may provide a stimulus that makes you want to eat.

Buy non-fattening food

Sometimes you may find it impossible to resist buying fattening foods. Packaging and displays in shops make it very difficult to resist. If you do buy fattening foods, such as chocolates or biscuits, put them away out of sight and out of easy reach so that you have to make a very conscious decision to eat some. Don't ever keep sweets or biscuits in the living room or the glove compartment of the car. Shop from a list and only buy items, which are on the list. The best time to shop is after you have eaten, it prevents you from purchasing greed-items.

Maintain record of eating habits

Some women eat a lot of their children's leftovers. Without thinking it through, they tell themselves that the food should not be wasted. Force yourself to throw the leftovers away and begin to give the children smaller portions. After work, if you go for a drink with friends, choose a small drink containing fewer calories, drink halves of beer, and don't accompany it with high-cal snacks.

Enlist help from others

Explain to your spouse and friends as well as colleagues what you are doing so that they can remind you to watch the calories, if you forget. Tell them that you need praise, not punishment and ask them to compliment you when you stick to your rules. Also, tell your friends not to insist on your taking more servings at parties or get-togethers.

Be sly but knowing

Use a little deception to make small portions appear large, for example, use a small plate. But be sure to measure out what you eat so that you know how much you have eaten. Don't put serving dishes on the table, to make it more of a conscious effort to get a second helping. If you are a fast eater, you might try coming to the table late to avoid eating twice as much as everyone else.

Know the six enemies: boredom, depression, loneliness, hunger, anger and fatigue

Boredom, depression and loneliness are generally problems for people who are overweight because they tend to use food as a means of fighting these moods, but you can fight these moods off in other ways. For example, keep a list of friends to call, think of starting a new hobby or joining an evening class. Make a list of things to do when you are hungry.

Some people who cannot express their anger find this inability makes them overeat. Exercise is a much better way of relieving tension and uses up calories. If you do not have a particular sport, try walking – an excellent way of relieving tense feelings.

When people are very tired they often try to get more energy by eating. You may be tired because you are not getting enough sleep or because you need to relax more in the middle of the day. As a rule try to get eight to nine hours in bed a day even if you are not asleep all the time.

Don't skip any mcal

Taking regular small meals can control hunger. If you skip breakfast and have a small lunch, you are bound to feel very hungry in the evening. Then you may eat a large meal, which more than compensates for all the food you have denied yourself. Eat three regular meals a day.

Have safe snacks at hand

Keep safe snacks such as peeled carrots, shredded cabbage, celery, or cottage cheese ready in the refrigerator. You can make the snacks more interesting by, for e.g., carving the carrots into shapes, mixing cottage cheese with fresh herbs such as parsley and putting it into a mould. If you know you will want a snack at a certain time, you can try saving one item, such as a slice of toast, from a previous meal.

Learn to eat slowly

Consider your eating habits. Do you tend to finish your meal while others are still only halfway through? If so, teach yourself to take smaller bites and to chew for longer. If this is too difficult at first, simply stop for two or three minutes, putting down fork or spoon. Avoid using your hands for eating. After the pause, continue trying again to eat small mouthfuls slowly. Some people put more food into their mouth before they have finished chewing the first mouthful. Make sure you avoid this. Research has shown that it takes twenty minutes after eating for a person to begin to feel full and to lose the feelings of hunger. If you finish eating within twenty minutes you will still feel hungry at the end of a meal. Try to pause between courses.

Increase the amount of exercise

It is important to take more exercise so that you burn up fat and food. Studies have shown that many fat people do not eat more than slim people but they do take a lot less exercise. Try to build exercise into your life even if it only means walking home from work or going up by the stairs instead of using the lift.

Choose method of dieting

There are two different approaches to dieting.

1. **The Cut Down diet.** In this diet you are given lots of information on calorie contents of foods and rinks, and advice on the right calorie limit to set and the right things to choose, and you are then left to devise your own diet.
2. **The Cut Out diet.** In this diet plan, you are given certain foods you can eat as much of as you like, other foods that are rationed and some foods, which are forbidden.

Research shows that both types are popular. Usually the Cut Down diet appeals to women and the Cut Out diet appeals to men.

Cut Down Method of Slimming

Average calorie requirements of men and women vary with their age and the amount of energy they expend in work and exercise.

Sex	Age (in years)	Calories burnt per day
Boys	5	1,700
Girls	5	1,700
Boys	15	2,900
Girls	15	2,900
Men	25	2,700-3,600
Women	25	2,200-2,700
Men	45	2,600-2,900
Women	45	2,200-2,500
Men	65	2,500
Women	65	2,200 or less

These figures are only averages and there can be quite a range of calorie requirements even when sex and age are the same. It is very difficult to measure total calorie expenditure directly on a daily basis. Each individual has to calculate his/her own calorie expenditure, based on the activities. Everything you eat and drink must be counted and also the calorie burnt in various physical activities through the day. Once you have some idea of your energy output, you must decide on a suitable 'energy gap' between your input and output. The size of this gap is your choice. Suppose you consider yourself a fairly inactive 45-year-old woman, you take the average value of 2,200 calories to be your energy output. If you set yourself an energy gap of 500 calories, this means that your energy input must be 1,700 calories; an energy gap of 700 calories reduces your allowed input to 1,500 calories.

Whatever energy gap you set for yourself, you will lose more weight in the first week than in any other. This is probably because the first energy reserves that your body calls on when output exceeds inputs are its starch stores in the muscles. Since these starch stores have quite a lot of water associated with them, you will lose quite a few pounds of water in the first week, as well as a little fat. The amount of water you lose will depend on the size of your starch stores, and this in turn will depend on your previous diet; a diet rich in carbohydrates fills up the stores. After the first week, it is much easier to predict the rate of weight-loss on a known energy gap because it is known that it takes a total energy gap of 3,500 calories to break down 0.45 kg of fat. So seven days on a 500 calories energy gap will cause a fat-loss of about 0.454 kg, on a 700 calories energy gap, the fat loss will be nearly 0.680 kg.

As far as calculating fat-losses and gains goes, all calories are equal and calories from any food or drink which is surplus to your requirements are stored as fat. So, a diet, which has just 1,000 calories, no matter what the food, will cause a weight-loss because there is a reasonable energy gap. However, it is particularly important that you should follow the general principles of a healthy diet when you are eating less, and this is why you should try to follow a few rules about the amount of fat, proteins and carbohydrate that make up your calorie limit.

It is recommended that not more than 35% of your total daily calories should come from fat and it is a good idea to apply this principle to your weight-reduction diet. Thus for every 1,000 calories that you allow yourself on your diet, no more than 350 of these calories should come from fat. Since 1 gram of fat contains 9 calories, this restricts the fat in your 1,000-calorie diet to less than 40 grams.

In the Cut Down diet, it is suggested that you stick to two limits, a calorie limit and a fat limit, because otherwise the counting would get far too complicated. However, do bear in mind that calories from sugar are 'empty calories'; they supply energy and nothing else, and so you should keep your sugar intake low if you want to stay healthy and ward off heart and dental disease.

To implement the Cut Down Plan, you have to know the nutritional constituents of each food element. Given below is a table to help you in planning your meals:

Description of the food	Protein percentage	Fat percentage	Carbohydrate	Calories per 100 gms.
Cakes and pastries				
Doughnuts	6.0	15.8	48.8	355
Ginger biscuits	5.9	16.7	71.2	447
Pastry, short, baked	7.7	33.4	54.9	548
Plain fruit cake	5.8	16.3	53.9	378
Sponge cake	8.9	7.0	55.1	308
Jam tarts	3.8	15.4	62.7	394
Puddings				
Trifle pudding	3.3	5.6	22.4	218
Jelly	1.9	0	19.1	82
Cereal and cereal food				
Biscuits, cream crackers	9.6	16.3	68.3	447
Kellogg's, All-Bran	12.6	4.5	58.0	311
Biscuits, plain	7.4	13.2	75.3	435
Rusks	6.0	8.4	81.6	409
Biscuit, sweet	5.5	30.7	66.5	556
Bread, brown	8.7	2.1	49.9	242
Bread, white	7.8	1.4	52.7	243
Bread, white, toasted	9.6	1.7	64.9	299
Cornflakes-Kellogg	6.6	0.8	88.2	367
Cornflour	0.5	0.7	92.0	354

Description of the food	Protein percentage	Fat percentage	Carbohydrate	Calories per 100 gms.
Custard powder	3.4	3.9	17.5	116
Macaroni, boiled	3.4	0.6	25.2	114
Oatmeal porridge	1.4	0.9	8.2	45
Rice, polished, boiled	2.1	0.3	29.6	122
Semolina	10.7	1.8	77.5	352
Soya. Full fat flour	40.3	23.5	13.3	433
Milk and milk products				
Butter, slightly salted	0.4	85.1	Trace	793
Cheese, Cheddar	25.4	34.5	Tr.	425
Cheese, Cheshire	25.8	30.6	Tr.	389
Cheese, Parmesan	35.1	29.7	Tr.	420
Cheese, Processed	23.0	30.1	Tr.	374
Cream, single	2.4	21.2	3.2	219
Cream, double	1.5	48.2	2.0	462
Milk, fresh, whole	3.4	3.7	4.8	66
Milk, fresh, skimmed	3.5	0.2	5.1	
Milk, condensed, whole, sweetened	8.2	12.0	56.0	354
Milk, dried, skimmed	34.5	0.3	49.1	326
Yoghurt, low fat	4.7	1.8	4.9	54

Description of the food	Protein percentage	Fat percentage	Carbohydrate	Calories per 100 gms.
Eggs				
Eggs, fresh, whole	11.9	12.3	Trace	163
Egg white	9.0	Tr.	Tr.	37
Egg yolk	16.2	30.5	Tr.	350
Eggs, fried	14.1	19.5	Tr.	239
Eggs, poached	12.4	11.7	Tr.	160
Meat and poultry				
Chicken, boiled	26.2	10.3	0.0	203
Chicken, roast	29.6	7.3	0.0	189
Lamb chops, grilled, lean and fat	19.9	45.0	0.0	500
Lamb chop, fried, lean only	22.8	25.2	5.7	341
Sausage, pork, fried	11.5	24.8	12.7	326
Fish				
Mackerel, fried	20.0	11.3	0.0	187
Prawns	21.2	1.8	0.0	104
Sardines, canned	20.4	22.6	0.0	294
Fruits				
Apples	0.3	Tr.	12.2	47
Apricots, fresh	0.6	Trace	6.7	28
Apricots, dried, raw	4.8	Tr.	43.4	183
Dates	2.0	Tr.	63.9	248
Grapes, black	0.6	Tr.	15.5	60
Bananas	1.1	Tr.	6.4	30
Cherries	0.6	Tr.	11.9	47

Description of the food	Protein percentage	Fat percentage	Carbohydrate	Calories per 100 gms.
Dates	2.0	Tr.	63.9	248
Grapes, black	0.6	Tr.	15.5	60
Grapes	0.6	Tr.	16.1	63
Oranges	0.8	Tr.	8.5	35
Orange juice	0.6	Tr.	9.1	37
Peaches, fresh	0.6	Tr.	9.1	37
Pineapple, fresh	0.5	Tr.	11.6	46
Raisins, dried	1.1	Tr.	64.4	247
Strawberries	0.6	Tr.	6.2	26
Nuts				
Almonds	20.5	53.5	4.3	598
Chestnuts	2.3	2.7	36.6	172
Coconut, fresh	3.8	36.0	3.7	365
Peanuts	28.1	49.0	8.6	603
Walnuts	12.5	51.5	5.0	549
Vegetables				
Asparagus, boiled	3.4	Tr.	1.1	18
Beans, French, boiled	0.8	Tr.	1.1	7.0
Beans, broad, boiled	4.1	Tr.	7.1	43
Beans, haricot, boiled	6.6	Tr.	16.6	89
Beans, runner, boiled	0.8	Tr.	0.9	7
Beetroot, boiled	1.8	Tr.	9.9	44
Cabbage, red, raw	1.7	Tr.	3.5	20
Carrots, old, raw	0.7	Tr.	5.4	23

Description of the food	Protein percentage	Fat percentage	Carbohydrate	Calories per 100 gms.
Carrots, young, boiled	0.9	Tr.	4.5	21
Cauliflower, boiled	1.5	Tr.	1.2	11
Celery, raw	0.9	Tr.	1.3	9
Cucumber, raw	0.6	Tr.	1.8	9
Lettuce, raw	1.1	Tr.	1.8	11
Mushrooms, raw	1.8	Tr.	0.0	7
Mushrooms, fried	2.2	22.3	0.0	217
Onions, raw	0.9	Tr.	5.2	23
Onions, fried	1.8	33.3	10.1	355
Potatoes, new, boiled	1.6	Tr.	18.3	75
Potatoes, chip	3.8	9.0	37.3	239
Potato crisps	5.9	37.6	49.3	559
Spinach, boiled	5.1	Tr.	1.4	26
Peas, freshly boiled	5.0	Tr.	7.7	49
Peas, canned	5.9	Tr.	16.5	86
Potatoes, old, boiled	1.4	Tr.	19.7	80
Potatoes, new, boiled	1.6	Tr.	18.3	75
Potatoes, chip	3.8	9.0	37.3	239
Potato crisps	5.9	37.6	49.3	559
Spinach, boiled	5.1	Tr.	1.4	26
Tomatoes, raw	0.9	Tr.	2.8	14
Sugar and sweetmeats				
Chocolate, milk	8.7	37.6	54.5	588
Ice cream	4.1	11.3	19.8	196

Description of the food	Protein percentage	Fat percentage	Carbohydrate	Calories per 100 gms.
Jelly, packet	6.1	0.0	62.5	259
Marmalade	0.1	0.0	69.5	261
Peppermints	0.5	0.7	102.2	391
Sugar, white	Tr.	0.0	99.5	394
Toffees, mixed	2.1	17.2	71.1	435
Beverages				
Coffee, ground, roasted	12.5	15.4	28.5	301
Lemonade	Tr.	0.0	5.6	21
Lemon squash	0.1	Tr.	33.7	126
Nescafe	11.9	0.0	11.0	90
Orange squash	0.3	Tr.	35.8	136
Pineapple juice	0.4	0.1	13.4	53
Tea	14.1	0.0	0.0	58
Alcoholic beverages				
Beer	0.25	Tr.	2.95	28
Cider, dry	Tr.	0.0	2.64	37
Cider, sweet	Tr.	0.0	4.28	42
Port wine	0.13	0.0	11.40	152
Sherry, dry	0.19	0.0	1.36	114
Sherry, sweet	0.31	0.0	6.88	135
Champagne	0.25	0.0	1.40	74
Chianti	0.13	0.0	0.19	65
Australian Burgundy	0.25	0.0	0.42	72
Beaujolais	0.19	0.0	0.25	68

Chapter **11**

WHAT TO EAT & WHAT NOT

Not everybody likes to count calories when they are slimming because it involves quite a lot of accurate weighing and measuring, at least in the beginning. Most people like to opt for a simpler system where they divide various foods and drinks into certain categories, and have specific rules that tell them how to treat the items in these categories.

People who use this method of slimming cut out carbohydrates such as bread and potatoes. That is an effective method of slimming but is an unhealthy way to eat. Bread and potatoes are good sources of protein, nutrients and fibre as well as being a source of calories in the form of carbohydrate. The aim of a Cut Down diet should be to do without the empty calories in sugar and fats and high-calorie foods such as cakes and biscuits.

There are three categories in the Cut Out plan, and the food and drink items have been placed into categories following the general principles of healthy diet which is low in fat and cholesterol and sugar but provides sufficient proteins, vitamins, minerals and roughage.

The first category is the one containing the unrestricted foods and drinks. All of them have a low fat and sugar content and contain relatively few calories.

The second category is called 'go carefully', because you must limit your overall intake of these foods as suggested. These foods and drinks are not alarmingly high in fat or sugar when eaten in reasonable quantities and they will ensure that you do not go without any important vitamins, minerals and roughage. If you eat high-fibre wholemeal bread and cereals you take in more bulk for the same number of calories and so should find your food more satisfying.

The foods and drinks in the third category are the ones you must CUT OUT completely. They are the foods, which are either very high in fat, or very high in sugar content, or sometimes high in both. Cutting out these items from your diet will do no harm whatsoever; in fact it should improve your health considerably.

It would be very surprising if this diet did not involve a considerable reduction in your calorie intake if you follow it carefully, you should lose weight at roughly ½ to 1 kg. a week (more in the first week), and your health will certainly benefit in many ways.

Guidance

Unrestricted

- ❑ Liver, kidney, heart, brain
- ❑ Poultry (not duck)
- ❑ White fish and seafood
- ❑ All green vegetables such as lettuce, cabbage, beans etc.
- ❑ Root vegetables, such as carrots
- ❑ All fresh fruit, except bananas and avocado pears
- ❑ Cottage or curd cheese
- ❑ Consommé, and low calorie soups
- ❑ Water, black tea and coffee, low calorie drinks

Avoid

- ❑ Cream
- ❑ Butter, hard margarine, fats and oils
- ❑ Cream-cheese
- ❑ Fatty meats like pork, ham and Salami
- ❑ Sugar, sweets and chocolates
- ❑ White bread (but not wholemeal or brown)
- ❑ Corn flakes, and non-wholemeal cereals
- ❑ Honey, syrup, treacle, jam, marmalade, Fruit tinned in syrup
- ❑ Dried fruit
- ❑ Crisps, savouries, nuts
- ❑ Salad cream, mayonnaise
- ❑ Rich creamy soups

Go Carefully

(No more than the indicated helping each day, and no more than four items from this category)

Milk	300 ml
Eggs	1
Meat	100 gms
Oily fish (e.g. herring, mackerel Sardines, tuna, salmon)	100 gms
Cheese	100 gms
Breakfast cereals (wholemeal)	100 gms
Bread (wholemeal, if not brown)	2 slices
Alcohol	1 normal measure of beer or wine
Soups	300 ml.
Rice (brown, if possible)	100 gms.
Spaghetti or Pasta	100 gms.
Potatoes	100 gms
Bananas	1 large
Avocado pear	half

Nutritional Requirements for Adult Men (vegetarian) per day

Food item (In grams or ml.)	Sedentary work	Moderate work	Heavy work
Cereals	460	520	670
Pulses	40	50	60
Leafy vegetables	40	40	40
Other vegetables	60	70	80
Roots and tubers	50	60	80
Milk	150	200	250
Oil and fat	40	45	65
Sugar and jaggery	30	35	55
Total calories	2400	2800	3900

Proteins 1 gm per Kg of body weight per day.

Burning Up Calories

By eating a 100 gm bar of milk chocolate about 660 calories are added to the daily total. If these are in excess of daily requirements, the length of time it takes to burn them off may make you think twice before indulging. If you don't burn off the calories, they become body fat @ 85 grams per chocolate bar. Exercises will burn off calories - but it takes longer than you think. To indulge in an extra bar of chocolate without gaining extra weight, one of the following activities should be performed for the time shown.

Activity	Duration
Walking at 4 mph	2 hours and 10 minutes
Cycling at 13 mph	1 hour
Driving a car	4 hours
Digging the garden	1 hour and 20 minutes
Swimming 20 yards a minute	50 minutes
Ironing clothes	2 hours and 40 minutes

Calorie Burning Activities

Even though we do not realise it, our body is constantly burning calories. Something as mundane as cooking can burn up 58 calories in 20 minutes. Here is a chart of some such activities:

(For every 20 minutes of activity)

- ❑ Cleaning/housework — 80-90 calories
- ❑ Cooking — 58 calories
- ❑ Shopping — 80 calories
- ❑ Dancing (moderate pace) — 80 calories.
- ❑ Jogging — 176 calories
- ❑ Gardening — 70-100 calories
- ❑ Mowing grass — 90 calories
- ❑ Swimming — 158-210 calories
- ❑ Typing on computer — 36 calories
- ❑ Walking (moderate pace) — 96 calories
- ❑ Walking (fast pace) — 126 calories

- ❑ Climbing stairs — 350 calories
- ❑ Walking down stairs — 120 calories
- ❑ Weight training — 110 calories

Facts about Obesity

Glands, metabolism and inheritance

Some of the common excuses made by a fat person run along the lines of 'it's the glands', 'it's my metabolism' or 'it runs in my family'. These excuses can all be considered together because they might all contribute partly to the fatness in some people (but not necessarily those who use them as an excuse).

Obesity due solely to the malfunctioning of one particular endocrine gland is very rare, probably accounting for only one in ten thousand cases. It has been said that the only glands, which are not working properly in a fat person, are the salivary glands, which work too well!

'Metabolism' is a very general term to describe the way in which food is turned into energy by the body, and studies of metabolic rate have indeed revealed vast differences between individuals, so that the amount of food they can eat without getting fat will also vary greatly. It has also been shown that individuals vary in their response to over-eating. Some will gain the theoretically calculated amount of weight when they are over-fed while others will gain less than predicted. What exactly happens is not yet known.

The fact that obesity runs in families is a well-established one, however, it is so difficult to differentiate nature from nurture that it is difficult to say how valid an excuse it is. The studies of twins and adopted children which are usually undertaken to resolve this nature-nurture conflict give confusing results, although there is a definite indication that some generic factor plays a part.

In summary, it seems that some people do have a genetically inherited tendency to fatness, which manifests itself in metabolic changes. However, there is nothing to stop those with a tendency to fatness overcoming it, even though the task for them might be harder than it is for others.

Childhood obesity

Recently, scientists have been particularly interested in classifying fat people according to the age of onset of their obesity. This followed some reports in the early seventies that the child- onset obese had more fat cells than the adult-onset obese, and it was inferred by others that the child-onset obese would have greater problems with slimming as adults. The publicity given to this theory, while being useful in prevention of infantile and childhood obesity, has been harmful in another way; being fat as a child has become quite a common excuse for adults who cannot lose weight easily. There is no truth in this excuse because it has never been shown that the child-onset obese cannot lose weight.

Puppy fat

Some teenagers and their parents use the term puppy fat to describe increased fatness during adolescent years. It is true that the changes in sex hormones during these years will lead to an increase in body fat in girls, but any over-eating during this time will lead to surplus body fat and this cannot be blamed on hormones.

Getting fat on the pill

Some women complain that they managed to maintain a reasonable weight until they went on the pill. Unfortunately there is no large scale survey which can validate this claim; usually, average weight-chances on different pills are given as zero as equal number of women loose weight on the pills as those that gain it. However it is known that pills that can result in weight gain can cause some fluid retention almost by about 3 kgs. If the weight gain is due to pills it is easy to identify the cause because as soon as the pill is stopped the weight gained is lost quickly. In case of weight gain due to pill, a change in the pill is recommended.

Getting fat during pregnancy

A lot of women will say that having children was their downfall as far as their weight was concerned. Here again, it is impossible to separate the physiological factors associated with pregnancy with the changes in lifestyle that usually accompanies pregnancy and the subsequent caring for children. A sensible weight-gain during pregnancy is between 9.5 to 12.5 kg. A weight-gain above the maximum limit will most certainly mean that the mother has added too much to her own fat-stores. Although it has never been shown that extra fat gained during pregnancy is different from normal fat, or that the mother's metabolism alters appreciably, some women find that they never lose this extra fat. Mothers who have a second child soon after the first might find it particularly difficult to lose the fat without a positive effort, because they lose track of what it was like to have a normal figure.

Giving up smoking

It is true that a lot of people do put on weight when they stop smoking. A recent American survey showed that men who had given up smoking during a certain five-year period had gained much more weight on average than men who continued to smoke. However, this only shows an average trend and does not indicate that a weight-gain is a biological certainty. There is no evidence that smoking alters your metabolism by an appreciable amount, and those who do gain weight are often very willing to admit that they do eat more when they stop smoking, probably because they feel the need to have something in their mouth al the time. If this is your problem, try chewing low-calorie gum. It is generally agreed that smoking is a greater health risk than obesity, so it is worth making the effort to give up smoking.

Middle-aged spread

The average weight of both men and women increases with age although there is no physiological reason why it should do so. More often than not, surplus fat accumulated gradually with age because of a gradual decline in physical activity coupled with perhaps an increase in food and drink consumption. Small changes in your lifestyle, such as taking the lift instead of walking up the stairs each time, can make quite a difference in the long term.

Ideal weight

An ideal weight chart could help to pinpoint the goal one has to work towards, although the ideal weight would depend a lot on the build and bone density.

Weight Chart for Indian Men

Height		Weight in kilograms		
Ft.	in.	Small frame	Medium frame	Large frame
5	3	48	54	60
5	4	49	55	61
5	5	51	57	63
5	6	52	59	65
5	7	54	61	67
5	8	56	62	69
5	9	57	64	71
5	10	59	66	73
5	11	61	68	75
6	0	63	70	77
6	1	65	72	80
6	2	67	75	82
6	3	69	79	85
Wrist circumference		Below 16.5 cm	16.6-17.7 cm	17.8 cm

Weight Chart for Indian Women

Height			Weight in kilograms	
Ft.	in.	Small frame	Medium frame	Large frame
	4 7	37	41	45
	4 8	38	43	46
	4 9	39	44	48
	4 10	40	45	50
	4 11	42	46	51
	5 0	43	48	53
	5 1	44	49	54
	5 2	45	50	56
	5 3	47	52	58
	5 4	48	54	60
	5 5	50	56	62
	5 6	51	58	63
	5 7	53	60	65
	5 8	55	62	67
	5 9	57	63	69
	5 10	58	65	71
Wrist circumference		Below 13.9 cm	14-16.4 cm	16.5 cm

Disheartening Factors

Some people, who begin dieting in earnest, give up half way because they find that their body weight remains constant after a certain amount of loss. This occurs due to a phenomenon known as the weight-loss plateau.

What is Weight-Loss Plateau?

Weight-loss is not a consistent process. It has been seen that the loss is maximum during the first phase and then tapers down. This phenomenon is known as the weight loss Plateau. It is a temporary impasse, which could put damper on most slimmers. But it is a hurdle that needs to be crossed without being psychologically frustrated about it. The body goes through three stages during the fitness effort.

The first stage – this is the conditioning phase during which the unused muscles begin to tone up and pains and aches signal this workout. Adrenaline and other hormones begin to get triggered off. During this phase, the weight-loss is minimal because the body is adapting to new stimulus and the muscles are not yet efficient enough to burn off fat. It is essential to continue the effort in order to reach the second stage during which there is more visible effect.

The second stage – during this stage the body that has already become conditioned becomes more responsive because the muscles have gone through the toning process and are vascularised. Blood vessels open up, allowing more energy-giving oxygen to saturate muscle tissue, which begins the process of burning up accumulated fat. The vascularisation builds up your stamina, reduces fatigue in the skeletal muscles and flushes out toxins from the systems. Exercising does not bring too much strain and the effort required is much lesser. The kilos begin to melt away and there is a joyous feeling of success.

The third stage – this is the plateau stage when the body begins to slow down. The pumping of adrenaline slows a bit, and the body's natural defence-mechanism compels the processes within to slow down. The weight loss becomes static and the visible changes halt. It is very easy to get disheartened and stop exercising. This is the stage that has to be dealt with patience and fortitude. The readiness to respond, the 'high' is effective only when sustained for limited periods. The body's natural defences and balance are merely trying to prevent rapid-exhaustion. The trick lies in recognising the plateau stage, which simply means that the body is gearing up for a fitter stage. It does not mean that the fitness potential is exhausted so don't ever make the mistake of giving up at this stage.

Chapter **12**

DETOXIFYING THE SYSTEM

Detoxification is the latest buzzward in health circles. The human body is increasingly coming under attack from various harmful and toxic elements in the environment, food and lifestyle. Everyday, new kind of chemicals and toxins are added to the environment, many of them still not detected. The toxins, unless weeded out of the system, can cause irreparable harm to the body.

How to Detox

To begin with, start including more fluids and water in your daily intake. This is really good to flush out the kidneys and will make you feel much better. You could even help yourself to some vitamin supplements. Make sure to finish your dinner by 8:30 p.m. latest, so that you get time to digest it instead of flopping into bed, right after a heavy dinner. This is a basic detoxification plan that will help you achieve some degree of relief from life's aches and pains.

However, if you really want to get serious about this, then you will have to make some adjustments in your basic eating pattern. Try these options for starters:

- ❑ Avoid foods rich in saturated fats like ghee, red meat, cheese and cottage cheese.
- ❑ Eat at least four to five portions of fresh fruits and vegetables in a day.
- ❑ Eat foods high in fibre like whole wheat, almonds, pulses and beans.
- ❑ Try eating white meats like chicken or fish once or twice a week.
- ❑ Try and combine rice, pasta or breads with lots of fresh vegetables. And try not to cook your veggies too much.

- ❑ Try and avoid caffeine-rich products like coffee, tea, alchohol and nicotine. You could even go easy on the cola drinks.

Smart Tips

Keeping a healthy, stable weight is one of the smartest strategies for long-term well-being.

There are no magic tricks to loosing weight. You have to have a sensible, realistic plan. You have to have the discipline to follow the plan. And you will have to make some changes in your lifestyle. In other words, follow the plan for the rest of your life, and not just a couple of months.

Take small steps. Do not make it extremely hard. Small steps often can reap big dividends in the long run. Since they are simple, you will have a better chance of staying with them long after the others have given up.

Here are some simple ideas you can use to control that bulge.

Keys to sensible Weight Control Programme:

- ❑ Stick with low-fat foods.
- ❑ Be easy on vegetables and fruits.
- ❑ Eat whole grains and beans for fibre.

Experts suggest that simple steps can a mean a lot when it comes to weight loss programmes. It can be made more powerful when you harness the body's mind-body connection.

1. Exercise
2. Trim your diet in mini-steps
3. Don't keep checking your weight everyday
4. Don't load on foods because they are "fat free"
5. Make simple changes in your cooking or recipes
6. Don't cut back on breakfast and lunch
7. Don't take too big a bite that you cannot handle
8. Double your measure when it comes to vegetables
9. Eat fruits for your dessert

10. Eat slowly - enjoy your meal
11. Be easy on your drinking
12. Tell your friends about your diet programme so that you can build up a support system.

Exercise

There is no substitute for an exercise regimen, for slimming. There are a variety of interesting activities that one can choose from, to accelerate calorie burning. Continuous, regular and effective exercising is the key rule for losing weight.

Trim your diet in mini-steps

A sudden and drastic cut in the diet is not an easy one to maintain so go slow and work gradually towards your goal.

Don't check weight everyday

Expectations of miraculous and sudden changes can result in frustration. Climbing the weighing machine everyday to record the changes might not show any. Once a week is enough to keep you going.

Don't load on "fat free" foods

Fat-free foods does not mean calorie free. Many people make the mistake of loading on the "fat free foods" and then find that they gained weight. Remember, 3,500 extra calories equal 0.45 kg of extra weight. This is enough to convince them that the dieting does not work and go back to previous unhealthy living style.

You can eat traditional favourites and at the same time shed calories from your diet and trim fat from your body by making small changes. For example, you can avoid 1,745 calories (enough to lose 225 gms) with the following simple tips.

Instead of having a strawberry milkshake made with ice cream and whole milk, blend four frozen strawberries, one-cup skim milk and two packets artificial sweetener. Turn the blender on high for about two minutes, until the strawberries are completely blended. Savings: 180 calories.

Don't cut back on breakfast and lunch

One of the big mistakes people do is to skip breakfast and lunch and eat a big dinner. This is not good. When you skip breakfast and lunch, you will end up in overeating later in the day. The problem with having a big dinner is that we are mostly sedentary after the dinner so there is no way for the body to burn off the excess calories; so they get stored as fat. When we eat breakfast and lunch, the calories get burned off for producing energy, as we are very active during the day. People in Mediterranean and Asia tend to have the biggest meal of the day at lunch time. The dinner tends to be very simple for them. This does make sense.

Remember the simple rule - When you under-eat, the next meal will make you more hungry. Don't compensate for a heavy dinner by skipping the breakfast and lunch. All it will do is to make you take a large dinner on the following day. The more you cut back, the more you're going to eat later.

One step at a time

It is important that we set up realistic goals when it comes to our expectations of how fast we can lose weight and what we can and cannot do. If you try to do too many things in too short a time you are apt to come up with disappointments that will mean to death of the whole programme.

Experts on behavioural modification say that it's too hard to make a long-term commitment. A one-day commitment is more manageable and easier to implement.

We can learn from what successful recovery programs do to make changes a part of life. The key to success is that it is much easier to break a bad habit or an addiction if you just focus for one single day on altering your behaviour.

Change isn't about making a giant resolution for a year but about making better choices every day. If you want to lose weight, you order salad instead of fries, walk to the store instead of drive, take the steps instead of the elevator.

Start with something really simple. Just do one thing positive every day—it may be to eat breakfast or take a ten-minute walk. Once you do it successfully you will be motivated to take the next baby step.

Double vegetables intake

Keep an eye on your portion size. Try to cut down on the portion of the meat and replace it with healthy vegetables and fruits. Instead of taking one serving of a vegetable at a time, take two—a cup of carrots instead of a half-cup. It really isn't that much.

Eat fruits for dessert

Instead of cakes and other calorie rich desserts, eat fruits instead. They are as filling and satisfying and tasty. Layer berries or peaches with low-fat or non-fat yoghurt or frozen yoghurt for a healthy parfait.

Eat slowly - enjoy your meal

Remember your mother told you to - "Chew each bite of food 20 times". That conventional wisdom still holds good. As it happens, there are a number of good reasons why thoroughly chewing food is healthier than stuffing it down.

Apart from the fact that medical research has shown that people who chew more slowly tend to burn up considerably more body fat than those who shovel it in, slower eaters also have fewer digestive problems.

Eating slowly will help you to enjoy the meal as well as to minimize overeating. Buddhists have coined "insightful or contemplative eating" for the practice of eating slowly and deliberately. When you eat fast, you may not realize when you are "full." The signal only comes later. You end up loading on the food in the mean time. Make your meal a social event by having wholesome conversations with your friends and family and watch what you eat.

Go easy on drinking

Another way to keep the weight off is by avoiding alcoholic beverages. Drinking a few glasses of sweet wine a day can mean an extra 6,700 calories a month, which can result in a weight gain of about one kilogram.

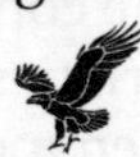

Chapter 13

WHAT IS GLYCAEMIC INDEX?

Dieting? You can stop counting those calories. According to a leading nutritionist, calorie counting is useless, because accuracy of calculation by the people can be illusory. Often it does not take into account the variation of the composition of foodstuff, nor the way it is cooked. In addition, it exposes the patient to a short-term deficiency in nutrients. In the long-term frustration and stress develops. Besides it has 95% failure rate after 5 years. The theory says that the obese eat too much and counting calories leads to the yo-yo effect on weight, i.e. losing weight and gaining again, leading to obesity.

The aim in a fool-proof diet plan is to include all nutrients and antioxidants and not count calories alone. A diet should also educate people of the composition of food stuff, mechanism of digestion and absorption of nutrients, thus encouraging people to eat better by making the right choice of food. e.g. 1 gm of protein/kg of body weight is needed or eat a carbohydrate with low glycaemic index.

In simple terms, a healthy balanced diet should include 50% carbohydrate, 30% of protein and 15-20% of fat. When you count calories one is bound to omit high calorie foods like oils, nuts, fruits like mango, grapes, banana and rice, etc., which are also an essential part of the balanced diet. Omitting such foods lead to nutritional deficiency.

What's GI

The jargonistic-sounding glycaemic index (GI) is simply a measure of the increase in blood sugar after the consumption of any food. The concept evolved out of the fact that all carbohydrate varieties do not produce the same blood glucose levels. When a person eats any food, it will finally get converted to some amount of blood sugar, and this is what is calculated as its GI. As with calories, foods with lower GI are preferred to those with higher counts. However, there is no fixed amount of daily dosage of GI required, but it is calculated with every food, in the sense that GI of less than 35 per food consumed will cause weight loss.

- GI of about 35 per food is ideal to maintain normal weight.
- GI of 50 -65 per food veers towards gaining excess weight in the long term
- GI of 100 per food, is an alarm signal and indicates high risk of obesity

(Since 1 gm of glucose converts into 100 percent of blood sugar, it is taken as the standard for measuring the GI of all other foods.)

The difference in GI

What makes the GI of one food different from the one in another food? The answer is not yet accurately known, though researchers are sure that there is more than one factor at work. Some factors are:

- Differing degrees of soluble and insoluble fibres in food
- **Starch in foods:** How starch in a food reacts with the amylase enzyme in the body will determine its GI, e.g. starch in banana and potato are a little resistant to the enzyme, which means they are not very easily absorbed, which in turn means that their GI is lower.

3% starch in ripe banana and 37% starch in unripe banana is not absorbed. As banana ripens GI increases from 59 to 90. 13% of starch from cooked potato is also not absorbed for the same reason.

- **Method of cooking:** When food is over-cooked it leads to gelatinisation, in effect increasing its GI, as in the case of rice, which in any case has high GI. Finely mashed food also has higher GI, thus whole apple, pureed apple and apple juice have different GI.
- **Individual reaction:** Not everyone produces or absorbs the same level of insulin, so, as body systems vary, so does the blood sugar in the person's body.

Does high GI food lead to weight-gain?

High glucose foods like refined carbohydrates increase the production of insulin, which convert to fat unless burnt. And guess what, these foods reduce the capacity of enzymes to break fat - which simply means, unhealthy weight gain. Any wonder why junk food has been flogged by dieticians?

On the other hand, there is something called 'lente carbohydrate', which is slowly absorbed in the body, and has low GI. In the long run, this is lot more beneficial, since the body is not subject to drastic levels of fluctuation in the level of blood sugar and what's more, they have high fibre content.

Thus food with GI more than 50 facilitates the storage of fats and leads to obesity whereas low GI foods like cereals, legumes, will induce weak GI and will avoid the storage of fats.

Link between diabetes and GI

For diabetics, food with low GI is very important as it delays glucose absorption after a meal resulting in improved glucose tolerance, whereas rapidly absorbed carbohydrate with high GI, results in sudden rise of blood glucose. The slow absorption rate of low GI foods in itself will cause lower blood sugar and insulin response.

GI and the digestion

The diet based on low GI reduces the amount of insulin secreted over 24-hour period. It aids in cleaning and flushing the toxic waste from the system and avoiding constipation.

Low GI foods improve even lipid (fat in the blood) profiles. In general there is a significant relationship between the rate of digestion of foods and the amount that reaches the colon. Rapidly digested food with high GI provides 1-2% of starch to the colon whereas digested food with low GI provides 20% starch to the colon. Thus foods of low GI provide increased fermentable substance to the colon, which increases faecal weight.

The delayed carbohydrate absorption helps in less free fatty acid absorption and reduces fatty acid level in blood making your digestion of the next meal easier.

GI of various foods

- Soya bean, peanut, apricot, leafy vegetables, salads, tomato, green pepper, garlic, mushroom have GI ranging between 10 – 20.
- Lentils, fructose, pulse, grapefruit, cherry plum, all bran, peach, green beans, brown rice, all dals, chana, vegetables except (root vegetable) contain GI varying from 20 – 30.
- Dried beans, legumes, lentils, chana dal, beans, apples, milk, fresh orange juice, apple juice, red wine, whole wheat bread, Chinese noodles, pasta, Indian corn, orange, dried apricot, nuts have GI between 30 – 40.
- Porridge, fresh peas, fruits have a GI between 40 and 50.
- The GI of Kiwi, brown rice, basmati rice, sweet corn, oatmeal, sweet potato with skin, banana, melon, pineapple, dry raisin with jam ranges from 50 - 60
- Refined flour, chocolate, boiled potato without skin, white rice, cocoa, macaroni, beetroot, cornflakes, honey, maltose, tapioca come under the GI of 60 - 70
- Rice flakes, roast potato, fried potato, white bread, biscuit, white sugar - 100, soft drinks (Pepsi, Cola, etc) have a high GI of 80- 90

Glycaemic Index of Food Items

Beans			
Baked	43	Black	30
Brown	38	Butter	31
Chickpeas	33	Kidney	27
Red lentils	27	Split peas	32
Soy	18		

Breads			
Bagel	72	Pita	57
Rye	64	Rye, whole	50
White	72	Whole wheat	72
Waffles	76		
Cereals			
All Bran	44	Cornflakes	83
Oatmeal	53	Puffed Rice	90
Shredded			
Wheat	69		
Desserts			
Fruit bread	47	Sponge cake	46
Fruit			
Apple	38	Apricot, canned	64
Apricot, dried	30	Banana	62
Banana, unripe	30	Cherries	22
Fruit cocktail	55	Grapefruit	25
Grapes	43	Kiwi	52
Mango	55	Orange	43
Pear	36	Pineapple	66
Plum	24	Raisins	64
Strawberries	32	Watermelon	72
Grains			
Barley	22	Brown rice	59
Buckwheat	54	Chickpeas	36
Cornmeal	68	Millet	75
Rice, parboiled	47	Rye	34
Sweet corn	55	Wheat, whole	41
White rice	88		

Juices			
Apple	41	Orange	55
Pineapple	46		
Milk Products			
Chocolate milk	34	Ice cream	50
Milk	34	Yoghurt	38
Pasta			
Macaroni	46	Macaroni & cheese	64
Spaghetti	40	Vermicelli	35

Quick Tips

- High GI increases blood sugar while low GI food is beneficial for diabetes, obesity, heart diseases and to maintain weight. Go easy on oil. Avoid junk food at any rate. When you take these precautions, you are automatically taking a healthy balanced diet, which gives more satiety value.
- All foods should be taken in moderation. Just because peanuts have a low GI, doesn't mean you can feast on them. You must eat a balanced diet that includes all food groups, then you can choose which food item you want depending on its GI and your need.
- An ideal diet that will help GI includes 8 fruits + vegetables in a day.
- If you want to lose weight, it is better to eat a raw fruit than to have juice because the juice is more easily absorbed and has higher GI. It will also make you hungry faster.

Eat Smart

Losing weight can be confusing, but if you start to incorporate the 10 Commandments of Weight Loss into your everyday life, you'll soon see big changes in the way you look and feel.

1. **Eat less fat:** Keep you fat intake at least less than 30 percent (some experts say 25 percent) of your total

calories. One gram of fat contains nine calories. If you cut back on fat, you'll control your weight, lower your risk of heart disease and boost your energy. Try replacing high-fat foods with nutritious low-fat options (like fruits, veggies and grains), rather than processed, sugary, fat-free snacks that are nutritional zeros.

2. **Eat less saturated fat:** Saturated fat clogs your arteries by increasing your cholesterol levels even more than cholesterol does. Keep saturated fat to less than 10 percent of your total calories. If you eat 2,000 calories per day, try to eat less than 22 grams of saturated fat. Beef, whole milk and cheese are all loaded with saturated fats. Replace them with lower fat cuts of meat ("Select" cuts instead of "Choice" or "Prime"), skim milk and cut down on the cheese.
3. **Watch your portions:** one common trait of obese is that these people load their plates with food. By simply cutting back on portions sizes you will be cutting back on calories.
4. **Combine carbohydrates and protein in meals and snacks:** Don't believe the myth that you shouldn't combine protein and carbohydrates at the same meal. These macronutrients work great together. Carbohydrates tend to give you an immediate energy boost, but the effect wears off quickly and you soon feel tired or hungry. Protein-rich can neutralize those feelings, keeping you alert and feeling full much longer.
5. **Drink up:** Water is one of the most important nutrients for your body. It cushions your organs, lubricates your joints, and keeps your skin looking good and transport oxygen to your tissues. Even a tiny water deficit can radically affect how your body and mind perform. You need to drink at least eight 8-ounce glasses of water a day (plus an extra 8 ounces for every 15 minutes you exercise).

Be sure to drink before, during and after every workout. Don't wait until you're thirsty to drink—that's a telltale sign that you're already dehydrated. Instead, you should check your urine. You should be urinating every two to four hours throughout the day. It should be clear to pale yellow (if you're taking supplements, it could be bright yellow after taking the pill).

6. **Buff up your bones:** You may think you don't have to worry about your bones now, but if you don't, you will definitely need to worry about them down the road. There are two proven methods for keeping bones strong and preventing osteoporosis:

   Get enough calcium and pump iron. Experts recommend getting at least 1,000 milligrams of calcium per day (twice as much as the average woman takes in), and some say that 1,500 milligrams is optimal. One cup of plain low-fat yoghurt has about 400 milligrams of calcium; a cup of skim milk has about 300 milligrams; and 85 gms of salmon has about 370 milligrams. Other calcium-rich sources include green veggies, such as collard greens, kale, spinach and broccoli.

7. **Eat early and often:** To keep from running on empty and help you control your weight, try eating four to six meals a day. Start first thing in the morning (after a seven or eight hour fast, you need to eat). Without breakfast your body has no fuel to function, and your brain and body are left running on fumes.

   Limiting your food intake to the traditional three-meals-a-day can cause wide swings in your blood sugar levels, which can also affect your energy and moods. Baby yourself when it comes to meals and snacks. What keeps most babies happy and cranky-free? Being fed continuously through the day. Eating throughout the day is also a great weight-loss strategy. If you're never too hungry, tired or cranky, you're much less likely reach for a Kit Kat bar. Eating large meals may also make you feel sluggish and groggy, because your body needs to shift extra blood from your brain to your belly to digest the food. Meals that weigh in at over 1,000 calories are not a good idea in the middle of the day or before you work out.

8. **Variety is the spice of life:** Varying the foods you eat will keep your diet nutrient-rich and your taste buds from getting bored. Studies show that tired taste buds lead to overeating. Keep them busy enjoying a wide variety of foods. Most people eat only 20 to 25 different foods, which strictly limits the nutrients you get. Even if you're getting a healthy balance of vitamins and minerals, you may be missing out on hundreds—if not thousands—of phytochemicals (substances in grains, fruits and veggies that appear to have important cancer-fighting properties). One simple way to add nutrients and wake up your taste buds is to try a new food every month.
9. **Eat more fruits and vegetables:** You may be tired of hearing that you should eat more fruits and veggies, but if you want to lose weight, they are a great calorie-bargain. People who have been successful at maintaining weight loss tend to eat more fruits and veggies than the average person. They're a key source of fibre, and they contain a wealth of cancer-fighting vitamins, mineral and phytochemicals. A diet high in fruits and vegetables can significantly cut the risk of cancers of the lung, colon, pancreas, stomach, bladder and ovaries.

   Stick to whole fruits rather than processed juices; a large apple, for instance, has four grams of fibre, whereas a cup of apple juice contains none. Whether you're interested in weight loss or simply want to maintain your weight and stay healthy, set your fruits and veggies goal at five servings a day.
10. **Eat more fibre:** Fibre will keep you regular (very important if you've recently made changes to your eating habits) and help prevent certain diseases, but it can help you lose weight. Fibre-packed foods (beans, grains, fruits and vegetables) tend to be low in fat and rich in vitamins, and they make you feel full! Insoluble fibres (found in bran, whole-grain breads, cereals and fruits) reduce constipation and may lower your risk of

colon cancer. Soluble fibres (apples, citrus fruits, oats and cooked dried beans) may reduce heart-disease risk by keeping blood cholesterol levels low. Adults need to eat 25 to 35 grams of fibre daily.

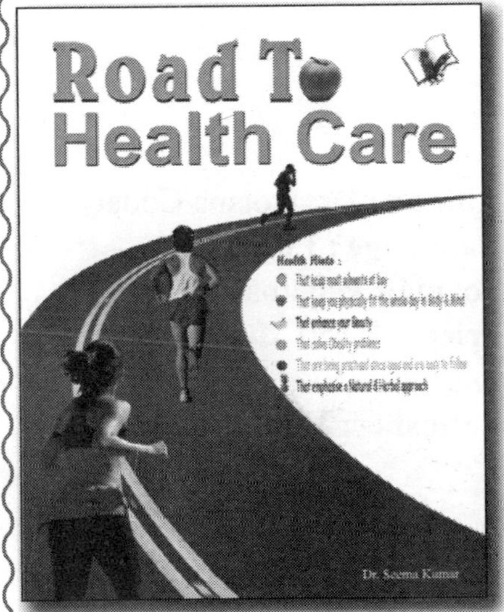

Author : Dr. Seema Kumar
Language : English
Format: Paperback
Price : ₹ 175
Pages : 176
Publisher: V&S Publishers

With ever-rising ground, water and atmospheric pollution, every other day one hears the name of a new disease. Ever since man began drifting away from Nature, he is falling into the trap of a materialistic lifestyle that has desensitised him. Today, we breathe air thick with exhaust fumes, eat processed junk food that has no nutritive value, drink toxic carbonated beverages and lead sedentary lives. All of this ensures that we are plagued with different kinds of problems at regular intervals.

This book shows you how to go back to Mother Nature to beat even the most troublesome and chronic ailments. With natural preventive measures that emphasise diet, exercise and herbal remedies, there are no fears of obnoxious side effects.

Whatever be your problem – diabetes, blood pressure, asthma, acne, menopause, obesity, stomach ailments, premature ageing or general complaints – this book shows you a safe, natural and enjoyable means to overcome it. Most of the ingredients mentioned in the book are the kind available in home gardens or off the kitchen shelf.

The book also includes hints for different stages in life. A separate section deals with varied problems in a woman's life through adolescence, pregnancy, lactation, menopause and general ailments.

Once you have read this book from cover to cover, you need not rush to the doctor every now and then, but will be able to take care of your own and your family's health yourself.

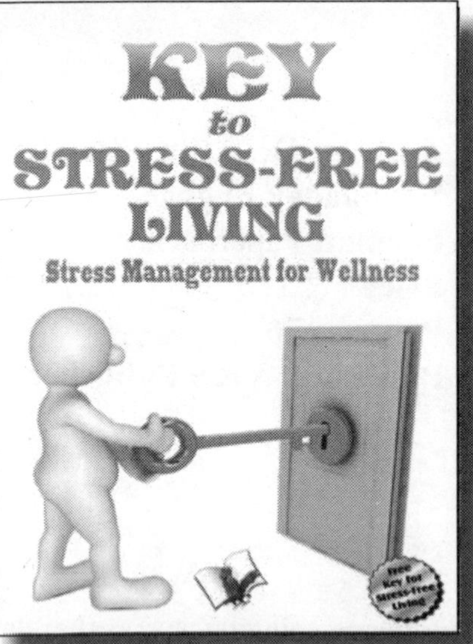

Free Keychain

Author : Dr. Jyotsna Codaty
Language : English
Format: Paperback
Price : ₹ 150
Pages : 136
Publisher: V&S Publishers

There are three primary aspects of life that contribute to promoting unhealthy stress which ultimately kills – inability to make decisions, feeling lack of control in life, and not having a plan or process in place to get to where you need to go. Spread over 18 chapters, this book has put together all the necessary materials to take control of your life, make wise decisions, and be proactive in taking care of things that typically stress you out. This book contains principles and ideas that will go a long way in reducing the stress that people have in this 21st century.

The fact that you are reading the blurb of a book on stress management, maybe out of sheer curiosity, signifies that you are trying to decipher if life could be made more meaningful and positive, no matter how contented or stressful life you are leading at the moment. This book is full of tips worth reading, especially given the author's credentials.

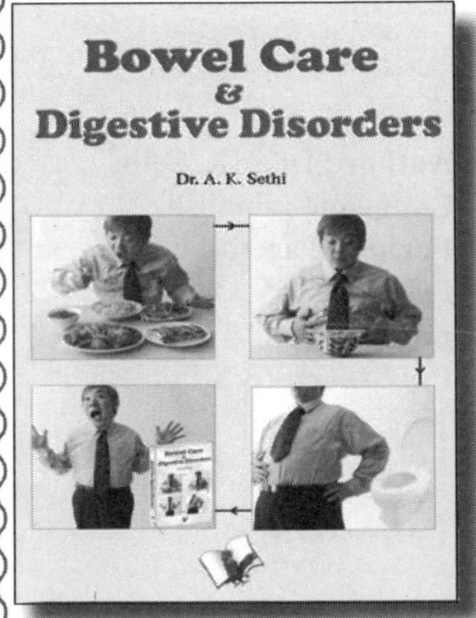

Author : Dr. A.K. Sethi
Language : English
Format: Paperback
Price : ₹ 135
Pages : 132
Publisher: V&S Publishers

Most people are shy about discussing Bowel care & Digestive Disorders, but few realize how important it is. The truth is that it needs utmost care and attention. The bowel has very few nervous leads- otherwise you would feel the digestion and bowel movement all day long. So, if you feel you have a digestive problem of sorts, you better attend to it immediately.

Most toxins enter our body through the digestive tract, along with our food and drinks. If we don't eat healthy, we tend to accumulate toxic wastes resulting in increased bowel transit time, and the wastes, instead of getting eliminated, stay put inside our body. These wastes, putrefy further and become a breeding ground for harmful bacteria and other parasites which in turn leads to more serious diseases and problems developing in the body.

This book is an authoritative reference source on bowel care and digestive disorders of various types. Written in a very convincing and captivating manner providing some anatomy lessons about the digestive tract, causes and symptoms of bowel disorders (constipation, diarrhea, etc.), the book lists proper diagnosis and treatment. It has been designed as an ideal self-help guide through yoga, meditation, ayurvedic treatment and alternative treatment methods like magneto therapy, acupressure, colour therapy, vastu, aromatherapy and music therapy to manage bowel disorders.

HOW TO HAVE SOUND SLEEP

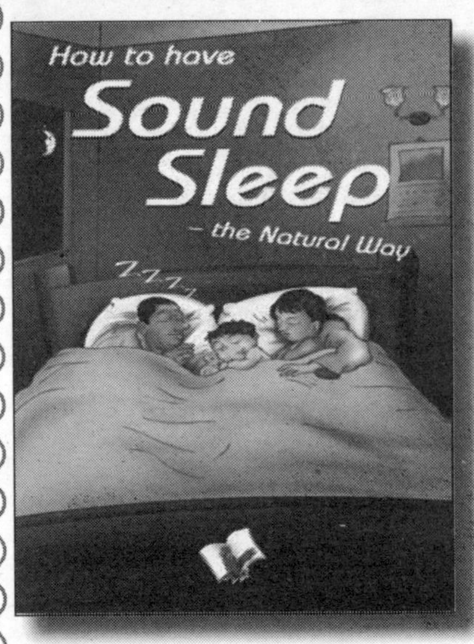

Author : Dr. A.K. Sethi
Language : English
Format: Paperback
Price : ₹ 135
Pages : 136
Publisher: V&S Publishers

Sleep Deprivation Can Make You Obese, Forgetful, Aged and Diseased for the Rest of Your Life!

Don't blame lifestyle for your disturbed sleep. Did you know that sleeping more or fewer than seven hours a day greatly impairs the production of thyroid and stress hormones. This impairment, in turn, not only affects the memory, immune system and metabolism etc., but also increases the risk of high blood sugar levels, hypertension (high blood pressure), weight gain, accelerated ageing, depression and increased risk of heart attack.

Researchers have also determined that sleeping adequately after a few days of disturbed sleep can very nearly erase any lingering sense of mental haziness and fatigue. In order to help you get a sound sleep and also to protect you from the need to take recourse to making up any lost sleep or disorder, the book details the importance, benefits, physiology and body reinvigoration of having sound sleep, untoward effects of sleep disorders and natural & non-conventional methods of managing it. Also explained in various chapters are advantages of proper exercise, yoga, naturopathy, acupressure, colour & music therapy, lifestyle changes etc., that enable waking up in the morning feeling fresh, fit and trim. A separate chapter is devoted to the Dos and Don'ts to highlight factors that contribute towards bringing sound sleep.

An indispensible book guaranteeing Sound Sleep to all readers every night!